Meeting
the Challenge
of Disability
or Chronic
Illness
–A Family Guide–

Meeting
the Challenge
of Disability
or Chronic
Illness
–A Family Guide–

by
Lori A. Goldfarb,
Mary Jane Brotherson,
Jean Ann Summers,
and
Ann P. Turnbull

·P·A·U·L·H·
BROOKES
PUBLISHING C⁰

Baltimore • London

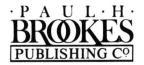

Paul H. Brookes Publishing Co.
Post Office Box 10624
Baltimore, Maryland 21285-0624

Distributed to the trade by:
    Liberty Publishing Co., Inc.
    50 Scott Adam Road
    Cockeysville, Maryland 21030

Typeset by Brushwood Graphics Studio, Baltimore, Maryland.
Manufactured in the United States of America
by The Maple Press Company, York, Pennsylvania.

Cover design by Nancy Johnston.

Library of Congress Cataloging-in-Publication Data
Main entry under title:
Meeting the challenge of disability or chronic illness—A family
guide
    Bibliography: p.
    Includes index.
    1. Chronically ill—Family relationships—Case studies. 2.
Handicapped—Family relationships—Case studies.   3. Problem
solving—Case studies.   4. Problem solving—Problems, exercises,
etc. I. Goldfarb, Lori A., 1959–   . [DNLM: 1. Chronic
Disease—psychology—popular works. 2. Decision Making—
popular works. 3. Family—popular works. WT 30 M495]
RC108.M44   1986   649'.8   85-19534
ISBN 0-933716-55-9

Contents

Acknowledgments

This book was inspired by the families we met and the research we conducted in several projects at the University of Kansas. Among the projects are the Research and Training Center on Independent Living and the Future Planning Project at the Kansas University Affiliated Facility.

We would like to acknowledge with sincere gratitude the many families who have shared their experiences and perspectives with us over the last several years. Special thanks go to the group of families who reviewed early drafts and gave us many suggestions for linking the ideas of this book to the reality of their lives. We would especially like to thank Eva Alley and Steve Alley, Rose Criqui, Velma Miller, Susan and Rob Tabor, Mary and Bill Reyer, Richard Ruth, Colleen and Max Starkloff, Shirley Young, Shirley Behr, Serena West, Lucinda Bernheimer, and Virginia Huguley. We would also like to thank Debbie Taylor for her contributions in the beginning stages of the book.

Editorial assistance was generously and competently provided by Connie Roeder-Gordon, Virginia Huguley, Susan Elkins, and Marilyn Fisher. Their contributions greatly enhanced the clarity of the final product. The preparation of the manuscript was made possible by the invaluable assistance of Mary Beth Johnston, Lori Llewellyn, Jean Roberts, and Connie Roeder-Gordon. We are grateful for the time and effort they devoted to the many drafts of our work.

It has been a pleasure for us to work with Melissa Behm and Paul Brookes from Paul H. Brookes Publishing Company. They have been sensitive to the content, imaginative in design and marketing, courteous in every interaction, and trustworthy in following through on commitments. It is, indeed, a pleasure to publish this book as a joint endeavor.

Finally, each of us would like to acknowledge the other. We have increased our knowledge of problem solving, communication, family dynamics, disability, and chronic illness. Most of all, we have been reminded of the power and pleasure of teamwork. The whole has been greater than the sum of the parts. We have invested much; we have reaped more.

Preface

A bout with the flu. A broken finger. A tonsillectomy. All of us have known the pain of illness or injury.

But, chances are, if you are reading this book, you and your family are facing a bigger challenge. Whether your father is recovering from a stroke, your sister is partially sighted, your child has Down syndrome, or your aunt has diabetes, a disability or chronic illness has brought changes to your family's life. The special needs created require coping skills beyond those demanded by the "ordinary" circumstances of life. How do you adjust?

This book will help you answer that question. It will help you tap your inner resources of strength and learn how to make the most of other resources around you.

Disability can refer to many conditions. These include physical handicaps, visual impairment, hearing loss, mental retardation, learning disabilities, speech and language impairments, and serious emotional problems. Likewise, *chronic illness* can be used to describe a wide range of conditions: asthma, diabetes, cancer, heart disease, lupus, cystic fibrosis, and many, many others. Each particular type of disability or illness has unique characteristics determined by numerous factors, including: 1) severity; 2) age of onset, that is, how old a person is when the disability or illness occurs; 3) limitation on independence, or how restricted one is in performing the activities of daily life on his or her own; 4) visibility; 5) prognosis, that is, the outlook for the future or the chances of improvement; and 6) the presence or absence of physical symptoms. This book, however, is not intended to address the specifics of any one condition. Instead, it looks at the *common* impact, or effect, of disability and illness on families—and helps you meet the challenges that will arise.

Our basic beliefs about family life shape the content of this book. We want to share our beliefs with you from the beginning:

- Families are different, but *they all have strengths.*
- There are no easy answers that work for everyone. Families are entitled to solve their problems in ways that agree with their values, preferences, resources, and priorities.
- Families have a wide variety of needs, and these needs change over time.
- A disability or chronic illness influences everyone in the family and creates special needs. Families are capable of not just surviving, but of thriving, while responding to those special needs.
- Families can learn to communicate and solve problems successfully. Half the battle is desire and the other half is know-how.

This book focuses on the act, or *process,* of problem solving rather than on the result, or *outcome.* Thus, it is designed to help you take advantage of and strengthen your own resources and then to apply those resources to your specific problems. This is a two-step process, and we have organized the book as such.

Part I, **Taking Stock,** will help you take an "inventory" of your family—that is, to identify your values and the resources available to you—and to further strengthen those resources. Part I draws on the advice and examples of many families, who shared with us their problems, concerns, and methods of coping. We hope that you can adapt their suggestions to fortify many of the strengths you already possess.

Part II, **Problem Solving,** is a carefully thought out process that is being used in a wide variety of settings, ranging from group therapy to corporate board rooms. Its popularity is based on its simplicity and flexibility. You may find that you already use some or all of the principles of the problem-solving process, but we hope the step-by-step method we suggest will help you find solutions more quickly to the issues you face.

All of the chapters in Parts I and II contain examples and case studies illustrating the suggestions we are making. You will meet many families with different problems and circumstances. The specifics of some of these examples—the type of illness or disability, the nature of the problem, the personalities and characteristics of the family—may be similar to your own circumstances, or completely different. We have found that the ideas in these examples can work in many situations, and we hope you will find them useful.

In each of these chapters, you will also find exercises you can use to try the suggested ideas for your own family. We encourage you to use these exercises. They are intended to help you understand and strengthen your own resources and to apply them to solving the problems that YOU have. We are not implying that there is one right way to do the exercises. You may enjoy working on the exercises as a family or as individuals. You may want to organize a special time to do them, or you may find that it is more suitable to your family style to try them out informally—around the dinner table, for example, or while driving in the car. At the back of the book, on perforated pages, you will find a second copy of all the exercises appearing in the chapters; you may remove these pages if you would like, to make it easier for your family to work with the exercises. We hope you will use the exercises as flexible tools for self-discovery and adapt them to fit your own needs and personalities.

All of us have a wellspring of strength that lies untapped until we are faced with a situation that calls it forth. Ordinary families, with ordinary resources, can survive the toughest of adversities and the bitterest of disappointments by finding this hidden strength. We hope this book will help your family find its strength in the face of disability or chronic illness and turn potential problems into positive experiences.

1

Introduction

Someone in your family has special needs created by a disability or illness. It might be your husband or wife, a young child, an adult son or daughter, or an aging parent. The disability or illness could be mild or severe, temporary or permanent, visible or invisible. But whoever the family member is and whatever the nature of the disability, this book is written for you.

Professionals who work with families are now realizing what you have known all along: The effects of an illness or disability reach far beyond the individual to touch everyone in the family. Special family needs shape the way you think about the world. They close the door to some opportunities and open others. They can organize the daily routines of life. For some families, the illness or disability is a source of strength, bringing everyone together in a sense of support and shared purpose. For others, the same conditions are a tragedy that pushes the family over the brink of despair.

We have set out, in our research, to find out why families react so differently to the presence of illness or disability in a family member. Over the last few years, we have interviewed many husbands and wives, mothers and fathers, sisters and brothers, and persons with special needs. In all, over 200 families shared their pain, frustration, joys, and triumphs with us. We did not deliberately seek families who were towering examples of strength and fortitude. They were selected randomly and varied tremendously in their makeup, cultural backgrounds, and values. The special needs represented were also highly diverse in terms of type, level of severity, and age at onset.

Despite all this diversity, the consistent theme among families was their success in handling challenging circumstances. Typically, families had worked out their own accommodations to some of their problems—accommodations that would not have been successful for others. Even with their successes, all the families were still in the process of dealing with other unresolved problems. Over and over again, we were inspired by the ability of these families to prevail over some of their problems, and to do so in their own unique ways. We found, even in the most troubled families, an ability to make the best of a bad situation, to survive the major crises and small daily stresses that surrounded them. We talked to parents who packed up and moved hundreds of miles, without a job and without a home, to find services for a disabled child. We found husbands and wives who, for years, had cheerfully carried the load of physical care and breadwinning for a spouse with a chronic illness. We met adult sons and daughters who worked constantly to make life easier for aging parents whose special needs would have otherwise left them isolated and without hope.

Yet, we also found that these same people invariably insisted that their behavior was "no big deal." In fact, many of them did not want to be singled out or commended. One mother, whose son was born with cerebral palsy, put it this way:

> A woman at work brought me an article in a magazine about a mother who had done all kinds of wonderful things for her handicapped child. And she said, "Ruth, this is just like you. I think it's wonderful how you have managed all these years." Well, it made me real uncomfortable. I don't think I'm so wonderful and I didn't ask for that kind of compliment. I'm just an ordinary person. I only did what any mother would do in my situation.

This mother's comment is precisely the point we want to make in this book.

Every family has problems, and strength lies in the know-how and desire to face and solve them. We believe that ordinary families, with the ordinary resources available to them, have the capacity to survive the toughest of adversities and the bitterest of disappointments. We believe that all of us have a wellspring of strength that lies untapped until we are faced with a situation that calls it forth. We concede that life is not fair and circumstances over which we have no control affect us all. We can, however, learn to control our responses to challenging circumstances and lessen their negative impacts as much as possible.

To be sure, we do not want to gloss over the difficulties and suggest that all families cope successfully. Nobody wants an illness or disability, and feelings of grief, anxiety, anger, and sorrow are normal reactions. Acceptance is not a process of denying these feelings, but rather of weaving the fact of special needs into your overall life-style and getting on with the business of living. Still, the journey to acceptance is a long, uneven one, with many twists and unpleasant surprises around the bends. The ability to cope is not innate; it must be learned. Some families learn it easily, but most learn it slowly and painfully. And some never learn it at all.

Disabilities and illnesses are not problems; they are conditions, facts of life—just like being short or being in a wheelchair. Conditions are not problems in themselves, but they may bring problems, or they may make other problems more difficult to solve. For someone who is 5 feet tall, the problem is not shortness per se, but rather getting a book off a high shelf. If the 5-footer is a 16-year-old boy, he faces the same problem as that of any other adolescent—learning to relate to peers— but his problem may be made more difficult because he is painfully aware of his shortness. For someone with a mobility impairment, the problem is not being in a wheelchair, but gaining access to housing, work opportunities, and community services.

Disabilities and illnesses both create new problems and complicate the problems every family regularly faces. For example, every family needs a clean environment, but a family with a member with severe allergies has specific environmental restrictions. Most parents do not worry about their children's survival after their death, but parents with a child having severe mental retardation must face the problem of finding someone who can continue the care and guidance after they are gone.

This book is designed to help you apply your own family strengths to solve the problems created and complicated by a disability or illness. The concepts we present are based on five major lessons we learned in our conversations with families and in our review of other research. These lessons are deceptively simple truisms about the general nature of families, as well as families with an ill or disabled member. *All families differ, all families have needs, all families are busy, all families change,* and *all families can solve many of their own problems.*

We want to explain these points in greater detail using the examples of six very different families. Let's meet the families first.

Paul and Margaret Ryders have a young daughter Melanie, who is developmentally delayed. Although she is 5 years old and should be ready to start kindergarten, her language and motor skills are similar to those of her younger sister Leslie, who is 3. Paul and Margaret have been getting more advice than they want from family, friends, school administrators, and Melanie's preschool teachers on whether Melanie should be mainstreamed (attend a regular kindergarten with nondisabled peers) or attend a class set up exclusively for kindergarten children with learning problems. Living in a small town, their options are limited. They want Melanie to catch up in her development and to learn as many skills as she possibly can. They question the amount of individual attention she will get in kindergarten. Will the teacher really be able to help her catch up, with so many other children clamoring for attention? At the same time, the thought of their daughter being in a special class gives them a knot in their stomachs. Would Melanie realize that she has problems? How would she feel about herself? It's bad enough that her younger sister is beginning to surpass her. To complicate matters, Paul and Margaret are not in a position to give up their jobs and need to be realistic about the amount of time they can work with Melanie in the evenings. School is starting soon, and they are feeling pressured to make a decision.

* * * * * * * * * * * *

The Martez family—Carlos, Anita, Maria, and Ana—left their Cuban homeland in the early 1960s and settled in Queens, New York to start a new life together. Carlos, a skilled cabinetmaker, was able to find steady employment to support Anita (his wife), Maria (Anita's sister) and Ana (his daughter). After Carlos's untimely death in the mid-1970s, Ana graduated from college and started working in the public library system. Anita and Maria spent their days keeping house and praying for Ana's success.

Anita gradually began to experience short-term memory losses; she would walk into the kitchen and forget why she was there or pick up the phone to call Ana and forget the phone number. She developed other symptoms—dizziness, headaches, and confusion—and was worried sick about her health. After several trips to the doctors, Ana was encouraged to take Anita to a city medical center for more extensive tests. Their worst fears were confirmed; Anita was diagnosed as having Alzheimer's disease.

For several years, Maria and Ana were able to care for Anita. As her disease progressed, she lost bladder and bowel control, became unable to walk, and was disoriented most of the time. Maria was losing her strength to provide daily care, and Ana had to work to support the family. Everything they believed about family bonds told them a nursing home was out of the question, but caring for Anita at home seemed equally impossible. They desperately need to figure out what to do.

★ ★ ★ ★ ★ ★ ★ ★ ★ ★ ★ ★

David and Sandra Daniels wonder what will happen next. They say the "black cloud got stuck over their house." David lost his job quite awhile ago and has been trying to make ends meet on his unemployment check. The check just doesn't stretch far enough to feed and clothe their six children. David looks for work every week and is feeling very discouraged and depressed that nothing is available. He wonders if he would have a better chance in a larger town 25 miles from his home. He knows that it's no use to wonder, because he has no transportation. His car needs new tires and a new generator, and there's no money for either. Sandra and the kids always seemed to make the best of a bad situation until their latest crisis. The biggest blow has been with Joan, the 3-year-old daughter who is the baby in the family. Sandra knew long before the doctor confirmed it that something major was wrong with Joan. She held her head and neck and seemed to have flashes of pain. Sometimes she would lose her balance and fall while walking across the room. Finally, the test results were in, and it was confirmed that Joan has a brain tumor. The doctors are talking about treatment programs of radiation and chemotherapy. The chances of survival are not encouraging, but Sandra and David must do everything possible. The doctors estimate that the initial treatment will cost $22,000. No insurance, no savings, no transportation, no job in sight. The Daniels have no idea how they will manage, but they know they must find a way.

★ ★ ★ ★ ★ ★ ★ ★ ★ ★ ★ ★

At 42, Ben Kohn's life seemed to be very much in order. His wife Marsha and their three children (ages 12, 15, and 18) were healthy, happy, and energetically pursuing their interests. Ben's business in a suburban retail store had been successful to the point that plans were underway for major expansion. Marsha was involved in several volunteer organizations and hoped to return to the local *university for a graduate degree in urban design. Then, out of the blue, Ben's life changed drastically. An automobile accident resulted in a severe head injury. Ben was hospitalized for 7½ months, during which time his prognosis seemed to roller-coaster from bleakness to hope and back again. Despite the intensive therapy he received, Ben is now paralyzed below the waist, visually impaired, has severe memory losses, and needs to start relearning how to speak. During the months that Marsha spent with Ben in the hospital, she began to realize that extensive family, home, and community preparation was needed to accommodate Ben's needs. What exactly were his needs, and where was she going to get the help? Where could she take him to get the best possible rehabilitation? What in the world were they going to do with the store? How were they going to manage financially? When was she going to have to go to work? How could she work and take care of both Ben and the children? What kind of help would the children need in order to adjust, and would they be willing to help her? The sudden life changes and constant reminders of the loss seemed worse to her than death. Marsha was beginning to realize, more than ever before, that she had to take charge. But how?*

★ ★ ★ ★ ★ ★ ★ ★ ★ ★ ★ ★

Stephanie Buonomo is a high-school junior with dreams of being a courtroom lawyer. She has been on the debate team for the last 2 years and has a natural talent for making effective arguments. A family joke is that Stephanie's debating success has resulted from all the practice she has had with her mother. The major source of conflict is that Stephanie refuses to allow her blindness to deter her from anything she wants to do. Geraldine, Stephanie's mom, is constantly anxious that Stephanie will get hurt or disappointed in trying to reach her high expectations. After all, she and her late husband had tried for years to have children before Stephanie came along. Geraldine always considered her their miracle, and protecting her only child seems so natural. It is nonsense to Geraldine that Stephanie wants to leave home to be a lawyer. She believes that law is no job for a girl, particularly a blind one. Geraldine wishes Stephanie would get a job and be content to stay at home like her cousins. Furthermore, it is increasingly difficult to live on Mr. Buonomo's government benefits. Paying for college is out of the question. Stephanie is realizing that a strategic battle with her mother is not getting her closer to applying for college. It only results in arguments, frustration, and tension. She recognizes the need for a new approach, but is at a loss as to what to do next.

* * * * * * * * * * * *

Sharon Pelosi and her son Shawn have established their life together. Sharon, divorced from her husband 5 years ago, has a steady job as a waitress. She is able to earn enough money to cover their basic needs, but has none to spare. Sharon worries about the things that all mothers worry about: Will her son Shawn be influenced by the "gang" to try drugs? Is he developing a sense of self-esteem and confidence? Will he be "down on himself" if he doesn't make the football team? Will she be able to send him to college?

Sharon has some additional concerns because she is a single mother: What effect will the absence of a male figure have on Shawn during adolescence? How can she help Shawn accept the fact that alcoholism, not a lack of love, is at the root of his father's infrequent visits? How can she deal with her own resentment and bitterness over the total lack of help from her ex-husband? What should she do when Shawn is obviously upset about her occasional dates?

But there is still more to complicate Sharon's life. In addition to having the standard "mother" and "single mother" worries, Sharon has some special concerns stemming from the fact that she has an illness called lupus. Lupus is a tricky illness; symptoms appear and disappear, fluctuate from one part of the body to another, and range from mild to severe. Some days Sharon even forgets she has lupus because of the absence of any discomfort. On other days, she can hardly muster the energy to get out of bed, and waitressing becomes a torturous endurance test. Pain, fatigue, unpredictability of the future—Sharon must learn to cope with problems she never thought she would have. What treatment is most effective? Are the benefits of her medication worth the risk? What does she tell Shawn about lupus? How can she prevent him from worrying about her? What will happen if she reaches the point that she can't work? What will happen if she gets to the point that she can't take care of Shawn?

ALL FAMILIES DIFFER

These six families differ in many ways—family size, number of parents, cultural backgrounds, geographic locations, values, available resources, age and family role of the person with a disability, and type and severity of the illness or disability. These differences have an important impact on how each family solves their problems. For example, Paul and Margaret Ryders strongly believe that Melanie should be prepared for an independent life-style in the real world of adulthood. Their belief influences their educational decision-making even at the preschool level. Geraldine Buonomo, on the other hand, is resisting Stephanie's push for adult independence. She would prefer that Stephanie stay closer to home and not take risks in the real world. The Daniels have eight members of their nuclear family, whereas Sharon and Shawn Pelosi are the only two members of their family.

Each family's situation is unique because of the infinite variations in membership characteristics, cultural backgrounds, and values that exist. Take a few minutes to compare your family situation to that of the six families presented. *Can you identify one similarity and one difference your family has with each of them?* Being aware of the uniqueness of your family helps you identify your resources and needs and the ways these needs can be successfully met.

ALL FAMILIES HAVE NEEDS

All individuals have needs, but it is clear that the presence of a disability or illness can increase the frequency and intensity of some needs. Ben Kohn's disability has created many new needs in areas, such as mobility, that he probably took for granted before his accident. On the other hand, persons who have more needs gain experience in learning how to meet them. They develop resources—personal strength and a support system of family, friends, and professionals—to help them.

An important aspect of family life is that needs are typically shared by more than one member. Sometimes, family members have the same individual needs, and then, at other times, their needs conflict. Stephanie has the need to go to college and law school in order to pursue a career; Geraldine Buonomo has a need for Stephanie's companionship and security at home. Ana Martez has the need to work to support the family; Anita has the need for constant care. They will be more successful in solving their problems when both family members' needs are addressed, rather than when preferential treatment is consistently given to a single member. All family members can benefit from having their individual needs recognized and considered. *Can you identify some of the needs of the various members of your family? Aren't they equally important when considered from each individual's point of view?*

ALL FAMILIES ARE BUSY

The demands made on a family and the tasks they accomplish in a single day are staggering.

Consider a day—almost any day—in the Ryders' household. From 6:00 to 7:45 A.M., *a minor miracle occurs if everyone remains calm and avoids irritation in the flurry of activity that must be accomplished—getting up, taking baths, ironing a wrinkled blouse, preparing and eating breakfast, glancing over the newspaper, negotiating with the girls concerning whether and how long they watch cartoons, taking out the garbage, making sure Leslie has the day's first dose of Ampicillin for the ear infection she had last week, cleaning the kitchen, making the beds, preparing a sack lunch, dashing off a note to the babysitter to remind her about Leslie's midday medicine, signing a permission slip for a field trip, searching for a lost glove, rounding everyone up, finding something for Melanie's sharing day, leaving the house 10 minutes late to drive Leslie to the babysitter's house and Melanie to preschool, giving the instructions to the babysitter, and chatting with Melanie's teacher. Is it a surprise that Paul and Margaret arrive at work a bit frazzled?*

Then after working hard all day, family life begins again when the Ryders each leave work at 5:00 P.M. *and each picks up one of the girls, gets a report from the care providers on the highlights of the day, and arrives home around 5:30 (it is at transition times like this that they are especially thankful that they live in a small town where distance and traffic do not add time demands to each and every day). Now, the great dinner race begins. Margaret and Paul head straight for the kitchen; working together with the help of their microwave oven, they have dinner on the table by 6:15. Because the girls are always hungry when they get home, they have a hard time waiting. This is usually the time of day when most behavior problems occur. The mixed sounds of whines and children's television provide the background for Margaret and Paul's kitchen conversations about their day's activities.*

When dinner is finally ready (and it's almost never soon enough), the Ryders eat, visit with each other, and share the tasks of cleaning up. It is then usually 7:00 P.M. *and the girls have 45 minutes until they start getting ready for bed. This time is usually saved for family fun—reading, playing games, walking around the block, swimming, or going to the neighborhood park. Then, it's the bedtime routine with all of its joys and resistance—getting pajamas on, making attempts to straighten bedrooms enough to find a path to the bed, brushing teeth, taking the third dose of Ampicillin, telling bedtime stories, giving a quick backrub, getting one more drink of water, praying for dry sheets, and saying goodnight.*

By now, it's close to 8:30 P.M., and Mom and Dad scamper to attend to their responsibilities—discuss the bills and review which ones have priority for being paid this month, worry about the ones that can't be paid, make out a grocery list, do two loads of laundry, repair a leaky faucet, mend the elastic in Leslie's bathing suit, and worry about which kindergarten class would be best for Melanie. Before they know it, it's after 11:00, and they go to bed. Busy day? Yes, indeed!

The other five families described in this chapter have activities both similar to and different from those of the Ryders. Your family, too, has its own special responsibilities and routines. ***Think of yesterday's schedule in your family and all the tasks you accomplished. Would you characterize your day as busy?***

The tasks that a particular family carries out are influenced by its priorities. One of the Ryder's priorities is to have enjoyable family recreation in the evening—a chance to relax and enjoy each other's company. This priority influences their preference for a school program that does not require them to tutor Melanie in the evening in order for her to keep up with her classmates. The tutoring would preempt their recreational time. They prefer that school be the place for Melanie's instruction and home be the place to unwind and enjoy each other's company.

Another influence on family tasks is the number of available resources. Who can help with different tasks? Neighbors, friends, babysitters, family members, and professionals are all potential helpers. Families differ in the emphasis they place on getting help and on their sources of help. Sharon Pelosi seems to prefer a more self-sufficient life-style. She realizes that one of her difficulties is accepting help from others, even when family or friends want to provide it. Because her and Shawn's needs are so extensive, she recognizes that it is impossible for her to do everything. Bringing in other resources is a necessity, even though it may be difficult to do.

ALL FAMILIES CHANGE

Changes can occur for many reasons, but perhaps the primary reason is the passage of time. The Daniels are concerned about the health of their preschool daughter, and the Martez family worries about Anita's elderly years. Sharon Pelosi, on the other hand, is dealing with needs associated with middle adulthood. Each stage of family life has its particular set of tasks, expectations, and concerns. The impact of disability or illness is different at each life-cycle stage.

Most people focus on their needs at the current stage of their life cycle and sometimes resist thinking about the future. In fact, one of the most consistent research findings is that families with disabled members tend to take one day at a time. Geraldine Buonomo's desire to have Stephanie stay home and avoid going to college and law school is based more on a short-term need for companionship and safety. She is not thinking about Stephanie's needs or her own needs 5, 10, and 20 years into the future. An inevitable fact, however, is that the Buonomos' needs will change. *Think about your family's needs 5 years ago, your current needs, and what your needs are likely to be in the future. What are the major changes that have occurred or are likely to occur?*

There are many reasons why families with members having special needs tend to take this one-day-at-a-time approach. Clearly, for many families, today's needs or problems are all-consuming. There is no time or energy left to anticipate future changes or to plan for them. Another consideration is the uncertainty of the impact of illness or disability. At this point, the Kohns and their doctors simply do not know how much progress Ben will make. The same is true for Sharon Pelosi; how lupus will affect her in the future is a looming mystery. Finally, the future can be worrisome, because of uncertainties about financial benefits, available services, job opportunities, and community living alternatives. Often, it is easier to focus on today and not let ourselves ponder the question marks of the future.

Families, however, can learn to move into the future with confidence by anticipating and planning for future needs. The changes that you experience do not have to be threatening. The problem-solving process described in this book can be used to handle the changes that confront you now and those you are likely to encounter in the future.

ALL FAMILIES CAN SOLVE MANY OF THEIR OWN PROBLEMS

All families can solve many of their own problems. Consider the situations of the six families described above. All of them will probably get advice from others on how they should solve their problems. This advice will come from a variety of sources—grandparents, sisters, brothers, aunts, uncles, counselors, neighbors, therapists, classmates, pastors, physicians, psychologists, teachers, hairdressers, bowling partners, and co-workers. Some advice will be welcomed; other advice will seem intrusive. Some will be shared in a supportive way; other in a reprimanding style. Some will be based on fact; other strictly on emotion. Each family must sort through advice, take what is helpful, and discard the rest. Advice-givers, as helpful as they are, come and go on a daily, weekly, or monthly basis. Families must ultimately take responsibility for solving as many of their own problems as possible.

The philosophy of this book is that you and the other members of your family are the key decision-makers about your own lives. As important as professionals and friends are, you and your family must ultimately decide what your problems are and how you can solve them most effectively. All families differ. Problem-solving approaches that work well in one family may not work in another family. *Consider some of the problems that your family has faced recently. How have you proceeded to solve these problems?*

Above all, this book is intended to build on the strengths of families—natural strengths to which some families might be so accustomed that they do not consider them to be anything special. All families—yes, we mean **all** families—have strengths that should serve as the basis of problem solving. An important purpose of this book is to assist you in identifying the strengths of your family and to suggest ways that you can capitalize on those strengths in solving problems. In this way, you can tap your own wellspring.

PART

I

TAKING STOCK

Families come in all varieties and forms. There are large and small families, families with one parent, families from a wide variety of cultural and religious backgrounds. There are families who live near (or with) many relatives and families who seldom even call or write their uncles, aunts, or grandparents. There are so many ways families can differ that it is safe to say every family is unique.

Yet there is one way in which we believe families do *not* differ: They all have strengths. No matter how disadvantaged, no matter how troubled, no matter what the disability or illness involves, every family has resources it can draw on to help solve the problems it faces. What are family strengths? They can be tangible resources, such as money and skills. Consider the McNair family, for example:

John McNair is a mechanical engineer. After he was paralyzed in a swimming accident, a colleague at work brought him a stack of books and articles about rehabilitation engineering. After studying them, John drew all his own plans for adaptive devices, and, with financial help from his father-in-law, had them custom-built. With these devices, he has become almost completely independent at home and on his job.

On the other hand, strengths can be intangible resources, such as spiritual or philosophical beliefs, determination, flexibility, or love.

Most people are not as fully aware of their strengths as they are of their problems. This is not surprising when you consider that we all seem to focus on unfinished tasks more than on jobs already behind us. Counting our blessings is a luxury for a quiet weekend afternoon or Thanksgiving Day. Yet, we need to learn to do more than appreciate our blessings; we need to learn to *use* them. Just as the corporate executive carefully surveys the company's assets before making a new investment, we need to learn how to assess family resources with an eye toward shrewdly investing them in the solution of the problem. Values are a keystone in solving problems. You use your values again and again as you decide which problems to solve and how you want to solve them.

Taking stock requires that you think about the resources you have available to you. Who is in your family? What are their talents? Which of your relatives, friends, or neighbors can you call on for help? How can you call on them? How can they call on you? Other resources include the professionals and service agencies in your community. How can you find out what services are available? How can you have access to them, and how do you use them most effectively?

We also encourage you to make an accounting of the total range of your family's needs. What are they? Here, we mean not only those tangible needs, such as money, meals, clothing, and medical care, but also the more intangible needs everyone has for recreation, socialization, affection, education, and a sense of self-worth. Who is attending to these needs? Which do you consider more important, and which do you feel are unmet? The purpose of Part I is to help you determine answers to these many questions that bear so heavily on your family's ability to make effective decisions.

Throughout Part I, exercises have been designed to help you think through and pinpoint your own family strengths. If you choose to do these exercises, we hope you will jot down all your answers, either in the spaces provided or on the exercise sheets at the back of the book. In Part II, you might find yourself returning to your inventory— of values, of resources, of needs—again and again as you address the problems you want to solve.

But most of all, we hope you will write down your family strengths because we are confident you have many. Look upon your family strengths as your record of accomplishments and as a wellspring, or inner source, that you can tap for future growth.

2

Roots, Values, and the Strength to Cope

ROOTS AND VALUES

Everywhere we go these days, we hear talk about values. Politicians tell us we must turn to deep-seated American values to guide our social policies. They list such values as freedom, equal opportunity, strength, free enterprise, and strong family ties. These and other values characterize the American ideology. These values (at least theoretically) guide our leaders as they make our laws and policies and as they take action in the world arena.

Similarly, every family has its own ideology: the values that serve as guideposts for the everyday behavior of each member. We hold values about which goals we should seek in life and values about the right and wrong ways to reach those goals. We might think, for example, that it is important to provide a comfortable and secure life for our children; other values, such as a belief in hard work and honesty, guide how we reach this goal. To make decisions more complex, we might further hold the value that it is important for our children to have a warm, loving home life with plenty of attention from their parents. This value affects the first goal because we cannot pursue making a living to the point of neglecting our children's emotional needs. Again, still other values affect how we organize our lives to meet both goals. One family might decide that the father should stay home and devote himself to the children while the mother should devote herself to making the living, even if it means she works overtime or at two jobs. Another family might believe that both husband and wife should work so they both can have some time to spend with the children. Values guide the selection of our goals for every aspect of our lives—physical, emotional, social, educational, and so on—how we weigh and balance each of these goals, and how we go about pursuing them.

We gather our values from two sources: our cultural heritage and the experiences we encounter in life. Our cultural background comes to us from our ethnic roots, our religious beliefs, our social class, and our geographic location. For example, some ethnic groups consider family solidarity and closeness to be of prime importance and raise their children to think first of family and second of self. Other ethnic groups stress independence and individual achievement and view the family as important only to the degree that it nurtures individual growth. Ethnic groups that have historically been the victims of discrimination and oppression hand down values from generation to generation that are designed to help them survive in a hostile environment. In a myriad of other ways, the values of our parents and their parents before them shape our family lives: whether children should be allowed to talk at the dinner table, how to discipline a child (and why), how and who makes decisions, whether we go to college or immediately to work, and so forth.

Our values, however, are not exactly like those of our parents because of the different experiences we have had. Values can be changed by momentous events that happen to us; for example, going to war or being laid off from a job. For example, many Vietnam and Korean War veterans have adopted refugee children because their experiences overseas inspired them to relieve, in some small way, the suffering they saw. Values are also shaped by more subtle experiences, such as a friend's opinions or an article in a magazine. For example, a book on nutrition might lead us to lay aside our old family recipes and concentrate more on salads, broiled meats and steamed vegetables.

Values also affect the ways families react to a disability or illness. For example, arthritis, multiple sclerosis, or an illness that imposes restrictions on physical activity might be more keenly tragic to a family placing a high value on participation in athletics than to a family valuing literature, art, and music. A family with a strong belief that children should be obedient might feel more stress with a hyper-kinetic or autistic child than a family believing that children's expressions and opinions should be encouraged as much as possible.

In addition to affecting emotional reactions, values affect the decisions families make about the actions they take. For example, Mark Jameson, born without arms and legs, remembers well the rules his father laid down:

> I had to put on my own prostheses by the time I was 4 years old. I had to put them on myself before I could go out and play. It took me an awfully long time, and I would sometimes get upset . . . . Sometimes my sisters would help me if we were in a hurry, but if Dad caught them doing it, we'd get in trouble.

Mr. Jameson's value, that his son should grow up to be independent, guided his child raising. But Mrs. Martin had a different set of values that guided the way she raised her severely disabled son:

> The doctor said just to take him home and love him, that he'd never be much more than a vegetable. So that's what I did . . . . It's OK with me. As long as he's happy and comfortable, that's all I want.

One set of values led the Richards family to do everything possible to find an effective treatment for Mrs. Richard's cancer:

> As long as there is breath in my body I won't give up. I owe Mom that much—she always taught us kids to never give up, to have the confidence that we'll win in the end. I feel that if I can be there for Mom, we can lick this thing together.

On the other hand, the values of the Carmichael family led to a very different decision about heart bypass surgery for Mr. Carmichael. As he put it:

> What's the good of having surgery if my life has to be so restricted afterwards? I don't call that living if I can't keep on going to work, meeting my friends, doing everything I do now. I'm not interested in a long life—I just want to live a good one.

Although values affect our reaction to problems, we need also to realize that a disability or illness can, in turn, have an impact on the values we hold. Many people have told us that the experience of disability or illness has changed their minds about what is important to them. For example, one woman told us how her husband's emphysema had changed her view of life:

> Before Jim got sick the kinds of stuff I used to worry about were things like how I was going to re-cover the couch. Now I look back on that time in my life and think how shallow it all was . . . . I guess what I have gained is a sense of what's really important to me.

The brother of a mentally disabled woman talked of the values he learned growing up with his sister:

> She taught me to be tolerant of people who are different. I don't just turn away from people who are a little slow; I'm more patient. I know if you just give them time they'll say or do something worthwhile.

Many of these changes in values are, in the opinion of these families, a change for the better. In fact, these changes are one of the strengths people cite: that a disability or illness has given them a deeper sense of values and a fresh view of the world. We seldom think of the positive contributions a disability or illness may bring, but clarified and strengthened values and a closer sense of family ties are often noted.

Given the pervasive nature of values, it would be impossible for you to list all the values that affect your life. It is possible, however, to think about values in terms of goals. What is it that you want out of life? Table 2.1 is a list of common values people generally mention when asked to state what is important to them. Most or all of the values in the table may be attractive to you. If we could live forever, we might be able to pursue them all. Unfortunately, our time is limited. As you clarify your values, the question is, which of these values is **most** important to you? Exercise 2A is designed to help you think about your most important values.

We hope you will keep your answers to this exercise and look back at them a year from now. As we noted in Chapter 1, families are always changing. Even values, which may seem so permanent, change over time. This is why clarifying values is a never-ending process. It's important to stop and think about your values periodically and see how they've changed. By understanding what your values are and why and how they have changed, you can reach a solid basis for directing your actions and tackling your problems.

COPING WITH STRESS

Our values lead us to goals in life and guide our actions as we reach toward them. In the process of working toward our goals, however, we

Table 2.1. Common values

—A prosperous life (wealth, beautiful surroundings, money to live without worry)
—A peaceful life (harmony and serenity)
—A balanced life (equal achievement and happiness among work, family, and personal life)
—An exciting life (stimulating, active, adventurous, willingness to take risks)
—An independent life (freedom to act on one's own choices)
—A self-sufficient life (taking care of one's own needs)
—A secure life (safe and protected from harm)
—A happy life (contentedness)
—A cheerful life (lighthearted, joyful, positive outlook)
—A fair life (doing what's right for everyone, equal opportunity for all)
—A broadminded life (accepting differences, willing to try new things)
—A rational life (a consistent, logical, problem-solving approach)
—A loving life (affection, tenderness, intimacy)
—A pleasurable life (plenty of fun and leisure, sports and other activities, relaxation)
—A healthy life (physically fit, good nutrition and exercise, feeling strong and well)
—A creative life (making or fixing things with one's hands, art, music, writing, sewing, crafts, mechanics, woodworking, etc.)
—A contributing life (doing something to make life better for others, helping people)
—A spiritual life
—A dignified life (achieving a sense of self-respect or self-worth)
—A recognized life (achieving social or professional recognition, respect from others, admiration)
—A life of friendship (close companionship and mutual support with others)
—A wise life (achieving a mature understanding of life, having a broad base of knowledge or education)
—A powerful life (achieving control and authority over others)
—A conforming life (minimizing differences between self and others)
—A natural life (living close to nature, preserving nature)

encounter daily irritations and major setbacks that put stress on ourselves and on our family relationships. There are everyday irritations that ruffle our composure, such as traffic jams, a tight deadline on the job, or a spilled bag of groceries. Some of us face daily insults and obstacles that are the result of poverty or discrimination or both. There are also major events that threaten us, such as unemployment, a flood, or a divorce.

Exercise 2A

1. List the *three* values that are *most* important to you in life. (Use Table 2.1 to help you get started in your thinking, but of course, don't limit yourself—what's most important to *you*?)

2. Compare your answers with those of other family members. How are they similar? Different? How do all your family values affect the way you live?

3. If possible, think about your life before there was a disability or illness in your family. What were your top values then? How has the disability or illness affected your family's values?

The actions we take to deal with stress and, indeed, the things we consider stressful are also guided by values. Over time, we develop particular *coping strategies* designed to reduce our feelings of stress. And because stress is a major threat to well-being whether it arises from petty events or critical problems, successful coping strategies are important weapons in your family's arsenal of resources. In many ways, the resource-building and problem-solving ideas throughout this book are nothing more than suggestions for adding to or strengthening your coping strategies. In this chapter you can survey the types of coping strategies you use now and consider how values dictate the stresses to which you attend and the coping strategies you choose.

Obviously, a disability or illness is itself a major life crisis, as is unemployment or divorce. But disabilities and illnesses also carry with them a number of side effects that cause stress to pile up. Families encounter rude remarks from strangers; they deal with thoughtless professionals or snarled red tape in service agencies. There may be an unrelenting demand for physical or nursing care or supervision of the person with an illness. And in the back of everyone's mind there is an undercurrent of stress—a constant nagging worry about the future, when parents, spouse, or children are too old to care for the person with the illness or disability. All this, in addition to the stresses most families feel—too many bills, not enough time to get everything done. Families with a disabled or chronically ill member need to know how to cope especially well.

Think about the last time you had a day when everything seemed to go wrong. What did you do to make yourself feel better? Some people take a long, peaceful walk in the woods; other people jog. Some relax in a hot bath or pick up a novel or watch TV. Some people buy something nice for themselves; others reach for a big piece of cake or a drink. Some people talk to a friend; others turn to religion. Still others stick doggedly with a problem until it's resolved, or try to put it all in a more positive perspective. Some people do several of these things.

Once again, every family differs in its response to stress. Even the things we find stressful differ from family to family. For instance, one woman found it necessary to take a break from the demands of caring for her mother, who had been confined to bed after a stroke:

> I had to arrange things so I could get away once or twice a week. I feel I am a better daughter when I am with her if I do that.

On the other hand, one sister of a man with cerebral palsy noted that her mother never felt any particular need to get away:

> I don't remember ever being left with a babysitter, even before Jeremy was born. Mom and Dad never were much for partying, and anything we did for fun we did as a family. Mom always liked to say she was just a homebody.

Experts have classified the many coping strategies people use into five major categories: *passive appraisal, reframing, spiritual support, social support,* and *formal support.* As we discuss them, think about your own strategies. Chances are that you have used most or all of these at one time or another.

Passive Appraisal

The first coping strategy is called *passive appraisal*—ignoring the problem or denying that it exists, perhaps in the hope it will go away. This is the strategy we use when we pour ourselves a drink or collapse in a chair and turn on the TV. It is also the strategy people often use when they are first confronted with a disability or illness. Renee Johnson, for example, did not accept the permanency of her husband's disability for almost a year following his return from Vietnam. Her husband told us:

> She couldn't believe I was never going to get up and walk again. She kept talking about miracles, or maybe new doctors. She thought the VA [Veterans Administration] wasn't doing everything it could. She would tell me we were going to go dancing next weekend, crazy stuff like that. I finally just had to tell her, "Renee, I'm in this chair and that's where I'm going to be the rest of my life." She just broke down and cried, but after that she was OK. Sometimes I think it was harder for her to accept than it was for me.

Renee's denial of her husband's disability served a valuable temporary purpose: It cushioned her against the shock and helped her gradually come to terms with this man who was in some ways very different from the one she married. The trick is, of course, knowing when to use passive appraisal and when not to use it. That is the moral of the well-known prayer: "God grant me the courage to change what I can, the serenity to accept what I can't, and the wisdom to know the difference."

Reframing

The second type of coping strategy is called *reframing,* looking at a problem in a different light in order to make it less stressful. Reframing might involve literally redefining the problem so that we can go on with our lives. For instance, one man told us:

> When I finally started thinking of my mother's memory loss and the pain in her legs as a disability, rather than an illness, I could stop resenting the loss and feel more empathic for her. I stopped a 15-year battle to get her to see "the right doctor" and spent more time talking to her, knowing my time left with her would be limited and therefore more precious.

There are many ways to reframe a problem. For instance, looking at the contributions of a disability or illness to family values, as we did a little earlier, is one type of reframing. Logical problem solving, which is one of the main themes of this book, is another. Still another way to reframe a situation is to look at it with humor. One father told us about his use of humor to remove the stress from taking his mentally disabled son out in public:

> It used to bother me that people would stare at Tim when we were out in public. Then a friend told me about a remark she used when people stared at her son . . . . The next time it happened, I decided to try it out. I marched up to a woman who was staring at Tim and I said, "You seem interested in my son. Would you like to meet him?" When she looked at me, though, I realized she was mentally retarded, too—and she said, "Well, yes, I would." . . . Now, when I see people staring at Tim I think, well, maybe they really do want to meet him.

Another form of reframing used by many families with disabled members is called positive comparison. This involves looking at other people's problems and deciding our own are less serious. Oddly enough, most of us would rather keep our own problems than take on someone else's. One woman whose father lives with her told us:

> When I see those other folks at the nursing home whose minds have gone, my heart just goes out to their relatives. They don't even know their own children sometimes! Pop is bedridden and crotchety at times, but his mind is sharp as a tack. The kids gather round his bed and he tells them stories . . . how wonderful they'll have these memories.

A father whose daughter is a wheelchair-user said:

> I'll take my own problem. I would not want to chase a kid around. We never had to pay for dancing lessons or Brownie uniforms. We never had to worry about her wearing out shoes.

And a mother of a preschooler with severe and multiple disabilities told us:

> When I see those children at the preschool with terrible behavior problems, I wonder how their mothers manage. They must be exhausted. Andrea just lays quietly, and she smiles at me. She'll never have to go out in the world and be aware that she's different, that she just doesn't fit in. She'll at least be spared that hurt.

Spiritual Support

The third type of coping strategy is seeking *spiritual support.* Many people find great comfort in prayer, meditation, reading the Bible, or attending religious services. For many people, spiritual support is a search for meaning in a chronic illness, an explanation of why it happened in a world where good people are supposed to be rewarded. A disability is a random, chaotic event, and a spiritual interpretation is often used to bring back a sense of orderliness and purpose to the universe. A father of a young man with cerebral palsy told us:

> I have always believed God has a plan for that boy, a job He wants him to do, or a lesson He wants the world to learn. It's my job to make sure Jeremy is able to carry out that plan.

People turn to spiritual support to give them the strength to get through a difficult situation. This was how the wife of a stroke victim found strength:

> The good Lord only gives us as many burdens as He thinks we can handle. He must think I'm a pretty strong person to put this much trust in me. I can't let Him down.

A mother of a developmentally delayed preschooler found her strength in an Eastern philosophy:

> After Christie was diagnosed, I was just devastated. I purely wallowed in my grief. Then a friend gave me a book by Alan Watts on Zen. It gave me such peace to think of the universe as a seamless whole, with Christie a part of it. In everything that really matters, Christie is as much a part of the world as any of us.

Social Support

The fourth type of coping strategy is seeking *social support.* Social support is practical help or moral support from friends, family, and acquaintances. Friends who bring over a casserole or watch the kids when we are in a crisis are providing social support. A warm hug, a pat on the back, shared tears, and a sympathetic ear are other examples of social support. Psychologists have said that it's less the concrete assistance we get from such relationships that helps (although that is certainly important), than the feelings of acceptance and self-worth we gain from friends who support us. A man whose wife is blind talks of the support he gets from friends:

We are friends with two other couples, and the relationship is just so special . . . . Christine helps my wife do the grocery shopping and puts the stuff away in a particular order so she can find it . . . . Quite often I'll come home to find my lawn has been mowed. Last week they built a new sandbox for Jimmy . . . . They don't do these things for us because they expect any reward. They do it because they're neat people and because they care about us.

Formal Support

The fifth type of coping strategy is *formal support*. This involves looking for help from professionals or service agencies who have the job of assisting us in certain areas. Welfare offices, mental health clinics, vocational rehabilitation counselors, doctors, lawyers, independent living centers, and public schools are all part of the formal support system. Most of these agencies are intimately familiar to people who have disabilities or illnesses and to their families. Some of them cause as much stress as they relieve. But a good professional or helping agency can be an important resource in solving the problems we face.

As you read the descriptions of the five major types of coping strategies, you might have recognized that you have used them all at one time or another. Or you might have found that you rarely or never use one or another strategy. How we cope, again, depends on our values and experience. One family may try to minimize the use of formal support because it values independence and "not taking charity." Another family may also shy away from formal support, not because of any firmly held value, but because of a bad experience with some professional or agency. Or a family might not seek social support because it values privacy and "keeping our troubles to ourselves." How we cope is a very individual matter. But no matter how we cope, we all do, somehow. And recognizing our own personal and family coping style is a step toward understanding where our strengths lie, as well as understanding our values even more clearly.

Exercise 2B is designed to help you think through the coping strategies you normally use. As you go through the exercise, think also about your values. What values lead you to find one coping strategy more effective than another?

VALUES AND COPING

By now, you should have made a good start at thinking through and clarifying your family values. We say "start" because clarifying values

Exercise 2B

1. Think of a stressful event that happened to you within the last 6 months. What did you do to cope with the stress?

2. Ask other family members or friends to think of a stressful event and how they coped. Make a list of the different coping strategies suggested.

3. Think of alternative coping strategies you could have used to deal with your stress. Which strategies would you like to use more in the future? Which less?

is a never-ending process. Not only do values change, but there are a myriad of different values attending every decision you make. We do not mean to imply that you should have a rigid list of values to which you carefully attend as you move through the day. Rather, we hope you begin to use your values to give you a sense of direction. Ask yourself what value lies behind some activity you are about to undertake. Is it important to you? Why? Will it lead to a goal you want to accomplish? If not, maybe you shouldn't waste your time. If it does, how does it fit in with other goals you have in life? How can you accomplish the life goals you want in such a way that the other members of your family are helped to accomplish theirs? Values are like the rudder of your family ship, steering it in the direction you want to go. It's important to keep your hand firmly on the tiller.

Similarly, your choice of coping styles should be flexible. This is a case of more is better; the more ways you have of reducing stress, the better able you are to cope with whatever life sends your way. In the case of the Kohn family, for example, the extent of Ben's disability is unknown for now, and it would do little good for his family to worry about how disabled he might be years from now. A little passive appraisal might be the coping strategy of choice. But in the case of the Ryders, Melanie's age requires them to make a decision very soon about her kindergarten placement. Passive appraisal would not be a good choice. What we hope is that, given a stressful situation, you will be able to recognize that you need to reduce those feelings of stress, think about the many ways you could do it, and then choose a coping strategy that works best for you *in that situation*. We cannot give you a formula for that—only ideas about the range of possible strategies that you can use to tap your wellspring of resources.

CHAPTER

3

Social Support—
Your Family and Beyond

The most obvious resources in your family come from the individual strengths of the people in it. It is easy, however, to take these resources for granted. If someone in your family is handy at fixing the car, for example, you might not realize how much money and trouble you are saving until you talk to someone else who has just paid a hefty repair bill. Even more difficult to recognize are the intangible talents your family might have. Someone might be especially good at understanding people's feelings and communicating them to other family members. Another might be a wonderfully cheerful person who can always make the rest of the family feel good about life. These are the kinds of talents that we seldom tally up as we inventory family resources. Nevertheless, they are a powerful source of strength.

Understanding the full extent of your family's resources is a two-step process. First, take stock of all the people available to you. This isn't as easy as it seems. Beyond the immediate family is a range of people—friends, relatives, co-workers—who provide social support. The second step involves thinking more specifically about the *ways* these different people contribute. This requires thinking about the range of needs of each person in the family, considering how those needs are met, and who meets them.

WHO IS IN YOUR FAMILY

When we say the word "family," many people think of the traditional nuclear family—mother, father, and children. Yet, more and more families today are establishing nontraditional households made up of single-parent families, gay families, or blended families. In addition, the traditional picture of the nuclear family has ignored other styles that have always been a part of some families, such as grandparents or other relatives living in the home or nearby. Nor are some people's definitions of family limited to blood relatives. One of the authors of this book has a close friend who has served as a grandmother to her children over the years and across the miles that now separate them. Your family might include a godparent, a special neighbor, or a boy- or girlfriend.

For still other families, a relative or ancestor who is no longer living is still very much a part of the family by virtue of his or her example or moral precepts. Memory serves as a source of strength, as in the case of the Cochran family. Many years ago, Mrs. Cochran died after an illness, leaving her husband to raise three preschool children, one of whom was physically disabled. Now those children are grown and on their own, and every one of them is highly successful and independent. Mr. Cochran says he found the strength to accomplish this task through the memory of his wife's courage during her illness:

> Whenever I hit one of the rough spots, or felt especially discouraged, all I had to do was think about her . . . . I would tell myself, if she could be so strong in the face of death, the least I could do was face this problem, whatever it was, the same way.

Beyond the people you ordinarily think of as part of your family, there are others with whom you come into regular or occasional contact. These people—friends, relatives, co-workers, neighbors, professionals, and many others—form a network on which your family can rely for help. Think of the social support provided by this network in terms of two of the coping strategies discussed in the previous chapter: formal and informal support. Formal support is provided by the many professionals who have been trained to help, as well as by the community agencies—schools, mental health centers, social service agencies, and health care agencies—that have been established to fill various needs. We consider effective ways to use formal support in Chapter 4, while in this chapter informal or social support is examined closely.

Members of the social support network vary widely for each family. For one reason, values define the scope of the network. Some families value the use of friends, neighbors, and relatives in helping with the demands of day-to-day life, whereas other families value "doing it on their own" and don't seek help from others. One father saw nothing wrong with turning to others for help with his 26-year-old daughter who was mentally retarded:

> We have a tight neighborhood and our friends and neighbors are all concerned about our daughter Chelsea. They have given much support with Chelsea's upbringing.

However another man, whose wife has multiple sclerosis, did not feel he could or should depend on others:

> I can't see how friends and neighbors can do any good. It's up to me. What can they do? Besides, other people don't recognize the problems.

Still another value—that support is the purpose of friendship—was reflected in the comments of a mother of a young child with autism:

> When I'm with my friends, that's when I can release my feelings and problems and be myself.

Her attitude contrasts with that of another mother, who had a very different value about the importance of not burdening her friends with her troubles:

> I don't talk to friends and neighbors very often. My son is not their problem. I wouldn't have friends very long if I talked about my problems all the time.

Your family's cultural background can also affect your willingness to use social support. For example, in some locations, black, Hispanic or native American neighborhoods have well-established networks to exchange goods and services with each other. Child care, rent money, furniture, food, transportation, and many other kinds of support are freely exchanged. Members of the support group who are willing to share what they have are given help from everyone else in the circle of friends and relatives. These exchange networks may have grown up as a practical response to poverty, or they may be a part of a cultural heritage. Whatever the source, they are a valuable resource for the families who participate.

Psychologists and other helping professionals have begun to recognize that social support has numerous benefits. Many studies have shown that social support is linked to reducing stress, decreasing physical health problems, and improving emotional well-being. One professional reviewed the role of social support in illness, hospitalization, pregnancy, childbirth, unemployment, and bereavement. He found that in all these cases, people with more social support made it through these crises or life changes with far less stress (Cobb, 1976).

A disability or chronic illness in the family can add a number of major and minor stresses to those experienced by other families. Social support can be an extremely valuable coping strategy for you. Calling on friends for help can be of critical importance when you are facing a major crisis, such as hospitalization. Still, it is just as important to develop and use a support network in your day-to-day life in order to balance and manage stress and maintain a sense of well-being. Although there are many professionals and service agencies available to help, they cannot do it all. Many people feel more at ease calling on friends whom they have helped in the past, rather than calling on professionals whom they have no way of repaying (other than possibly with money).

The social support network can provide three types of help to families: 1) material support, 2) emotional support, and 3) referral and information. *Material support* is self-explanatory. It consists of goods and services provided to the family. For example, someone might give you a specialized feeding utensil or pass along a used wheelchair. Someone else might help out with transportation or babysitting. We receive *emotional support* when friends listen to our problems with a sympathetic ear, give us a pat on the back, or otherwise let us know they care. Emotional support lets us know we are valued and esteemed and are a part of a network of mutual obligation and communication. For many of us, this sense of belonging is far more important than the exchange of materials and services. Friends can also provide emotional support by helping you maintain an active social life. Just having people to relax and socialize with is important if you are feeling depressed or overwhelmed.

The third type of social support, *referral and information*, is also important. By referral and information, we do not mean advice, which may be less than welcome. Rather, we mean information and options about where to go for help for certain kinds of problems. People who have already experienced a similar situation can tell you what agency is the best source of aid, who is the best doctor, or how to talk to a particular teacher. They can also share some of their own experiences—what they told their other children when their disabled child was born, how they managed social events where their disabled husband or wife was invited, or how they told their children that their mother was dying. These people have been in the same or a similar situation as yours, and their help can be invaluable. You no doubt have experiences you can share with others. One mother of a 26-year-old man with mental retardation told us:

> Every now and then, we old-timers are asked to be on parent panels to answer questions for the younger parents. They always seem so pleased and interested to hear how we arrived at some of our decisions.

Some service agencies have formed support groups where this type of information can be exchanged. In addition, through your doctor, the hospital, or the school, you can find people who share some of your same problems. Remember, just as in the case of exchanging material and emotional support, information and referral is a two-way street. You have insights and experiences that can be as valuable to others as theirs are to you.

We hope it is now clear to you that, for many families, the boundary between who is inside the family and who is outside the family is not always clear. And, perhaps, it is not so important to make that distinction. What is important, however, is that your inventory of family resources includes all the people you know who can be helpful to you. Exercise 3A is a guide to making such an inventory.

After completing Exercise 3A, do any of your responses surprise you? Are there any relationships between the members of your present support network that you would like to change? How would you go about changing them? The following sections discuss some of the roadblocks to building social support and provide suggestions for building and maintaining support.

ROADBLOCKS TO DEVELOPING SOCIAL SUPPORT

Developing and maintaining a social support network isn't always easy. There are many roadblocks that can confront a family. Here are a few:

Time

Limited time is an important issue in most families, but it may be even more so in families with children or adults who have disabilities or are chronically ill. The amount of time needed to care for a person with a disability or chronic illness, as well as to attend to the needs of other family members, often leaves little in the way of leisure time for developing friendships. Quality friendships take time and effort. Also, many friendships are based largely on sharing common interests. Sometimes a family may be so preoccupied with problems surrounding the disability or illness that it has little opportunity to develop outside interests on which to base friendships. As a result, many families with disabled or chronically ill members tend to feel isolated.

Building and using a support system takes time to coordinate—extra time that is hard to come by. Time invested on the front end, however, can save time in the long run. For example, setting up a neighborhood car pool for transportation may take several hours and many phone calls, but once it is set up, transportation needs can be met regularly for several weeks or months.

Stigma

Some families avoid building and using a support network because they fear the real possibility of stigma or social rejection. This can be especially true if a person with a disability or chronic illness has

---

Exercise 3A

1. List everyone whom you consider to be a part of your family.

2. List other relatives, close friends, neighbors, co-workers, church or synagogue members, and others who provide you with social support.

(continued)

Exercise 3A
(continued)

3. Listed below are several types of people who might make up your
   social support network, along with a scale to rate how helpful they are.
   Circle the number that best describes how helpful each one is to you.
   Leave the space blank if that person or group does not apply to you. Use
   a different color pen for each family member who fills this out, and
   compare your answers.

Family support scale

	Not at all helpful	Some-times helpful	Gener-ally helpful	Very helpful	Extremely helpful
1. My parents	0	1	2	3	4
2. My spouse's parents	0	1	2	3	4
3. My relatives/kin	0	1	2	3	4
4. My spouse's relatives/ kin	0	1	2	3	4
5. Husband or wife	0	1	2	3	4
6. My friends	0	1	2	3	4
7. My spouse's friends	0	1	2	3	4
8. My own children	0	1	2	3	4
9. Other parents	0	1	2	3	4
10. My family physician	0	1	2	3	4
11. Co-workers	0	1	2	3	4
12. Parent, spouse, or other self-help groups	0	1	2	3	4
13. School (teachers, therapists, psychologists, etc.)	0	1	2	3	4
14. Professional agencies (public health, social services, respite care, activity programs)	0	1	2	3	4
15. Civic groups/clubs	0	1	2	3	4
16. Clergy and congre-gation of your place of worship	0	1	2	3	4

behavior problems or visible symptoms that draw unwanted attention
or pity. For example, a friend might ask you to join him on a garage sale
hunt for some needed items, but you feel that taking a child with
behavior problems from house to house just creates too many stares
and comments. This may not only be stigmatizing to you, but also to

your friend. Stigma can increase as a disabled child grows older, causing even greater isolation for some families. Taking a severely disabled 4-year-old child to the park might draw fewer stares than taking a severely disabled 24-year-old adult to the park.

When the family member who is disabled or chronically ill is a spouse, stigma might greatly reduce the couple's social opportunities with their friends. For example, one wife of a husband with a physical disability commented:

> We just aren't invited very often to other people's homes. I don't think they are comfortable with having a disabled person in their house.

Many of these same concerns apply to families with a chronically ill member. A chronic illness that creates high visibility, such as baldness from chemotherapy or a puffy face from steroid drugs, often increases the stigma a family faces in the community. One mother of a son with chronic illness stated that stigma is also related to prognosis. She felt that chronic illnesses that do not necessarily lead to death, such as diabetes, asthma, or epilepsy, can be less stigmatizing than often fatal illnesses, such as leukemia or cystic fibrosis.

An additional source of stigma for persons with chronic illness involves the flare-up of visible symptoms; sometimes they are present and sometimes they are not. Some persons in the social support system of families experiencing chronic illness may think they are "fickle friends," not realizing that during times of visible flare-ups of symptoms the family may prefer to stay home, rather than deal with stares, questions, and concerns in social situations. If stigma is an issue for you and your family, you may want to refer to the tips listed in Table 3.1.

Loss of Privacy

Some families do not use social support because they resent the invasion of their privacy. For example, having a friend or relative come in to help with the bathing and dressing of a young adult with a disability or chronic illness can interfere with the morning and evening privacy of other family members, particularly if a family shares one bathroom. And what about the personal privacy of the person with an illness or disability; what are their preferences for privacy? When the loss of privacy affects the personal privacy of the disabled or chronically-ill person, then his or her choices should direct the decision making of how and when to use social support. Maybe the person would prefer only one bath a week to the loss of privacy

Table 3.1. Tips for coping with stigma

1. Discuss with family members what stigma means and when they have felt it. Have each person give an example.
2. Realize that people may hold prejudices, stare, or comment insensitively out of ignorance and unfamiliarity rather than malice.
3. Help to educate others about the facts so that they can learn to see beyond their fears and appreciate the person with disability or chronic illness.
4. Realize that stigma, like beauty, is subjective. Determine where it is a real issue and where it has simply become an imagined fear.
5. Determine if the threat of stigma alters your family's range of activities. Decide whether you are willing to sacrifice your freedom for the misperceptions of others.
6. Practice ways to respond to someone who says, "Ugh, what's wrong with him?"
7. Try using humor to put others at ease. For example, to the person who pities your baldness as a result of chemotherapy: "I told Jack we had to stop using that shampoo."

experienced by more regular bathing. Loss of personal privacy can lead to a loss of personal dignity.

Time, stigma, and loss of privacy are three practical roadblocks people often mention in regard to using social support. In addition, some of the values we discussed earlier may lead families away from using social support. However, those values need not be roadblocks. For instance, two families can hold the same value that they should be responsible for the care of their family member with a disability or chronic illness. One family can interpret that to mean they shouldn't accept help from others. But the other family might interpret that value to mean that they must ultimately be the case managers, orchestrating what other people do to help. It is possible, then, for some families to accept help and, at the same time, value self-sufficiency and independence.

What are some of your own practical and value-based roadblocks? Exercise 3B is designed to help you think through these issues.

BUILDING AND MAINTAINING SOCIAL SUPPORT

This chapter has focused on identifying all the people, inside and outside your family, who can be of help to you: family members,

Exercise 3B

1. Think about the roadblocks that you have to using friends, neighbors, and relatives for social support. We have listed a few in the text, but include any others that are specific to your family.

2. Now divide those roadblocks into two groups: those that are practical roadblocks, such as lack of time or transportation, and those that are value roadblocks, such as believing you have sole responsibility or that you do not want to burden others. List your roadblocks under each category.

   Practical roadblocks   **Value roadblocks**

3. Select one roadblock from each group, and list steps you could use to overcome that roadblock. Discuss your steps with other family members.

   Practical roadblock   **Value roadblock**

   _____   _____

   Steps: Steps:

including yourself; other relatives; friends; co-workers; neighbors; and church, temple, or synagogue members. Use these three suggestions if you choose to expand and maintain your social support network.

—Address the need for information on disability or chronic illness that many relatives and friends have.
—Practice reciprocity; to ask someone for support, you must be willing to give support.
—Help friends and relatives recognize the strengths and positive contributions of the family member with a disability or chronic illness.

Need for Information

Many friends, relatives, and neighbors of families with disabled or chronically ill members have some of the same problems other people have with illness or disability. They lack information and experience with these persons. Sometimes they don't know how to talk or interact with them. As one mother of a young man with Down syndrome commented:

> I don't need pity, I need help. If friends and relatives had more information they could see mentally retarded people are real people with real needs . . . . They should get the same opportunities as normal people. They should know how to be around handicapped people, what to expect of them and not put them in a corner and label them.

Think about the different roles that extended family members and friends play in many families. They take family members to ballgames or movies, provide a sounding board for feedback, invite family members over for dinner, watch the children while you run to the store, and help with the physical care of young children or infants. These are only a few of the ways that friends and family help in meeting the needs of others in their support group. Yet, with a child or adult who is disabled or chronically ill, a lack of information or fear of stigma may keep these persons from filling the roles or meeting many of the needs they do in other families. One grandmother expressed her fears concerning her son's new 12-year-old step-daughter with cerebral palsy:

> She wants to spend time with me and I would like to because she's a sweet girl. But I'm afraid I would hurt her. I'm afraid I would break her bones or

dislocate her shoulder trying to help her get dressed or seat her in a chair. I don't know what to do.

Sometimes family members might not understand why their friends and relatives have difficulty being around or helping the family member with a chronic illness or disability. The remarks of one sibling of a sister with leukemia poignantly illustrate this concern:

> We lived in the country far from town, so for us to get together with friends and relatives we would go visiting. But when my sister got sick no one came to our house and no one invited us to theirs. At the funeral so many people came with food and condolences . . . . And I didn't understand why they would help us at her death and not all those years she was sick.

Often, friends and relatives just don't know how to offer the help they want to contribute. Many would like more information if they could get it. One mother of a son with chronic mental illness said, "It took us years to get information on mental illness and our daughter is a psychiatric social worker!" Fortunately, more information and support are becoming available for friends and relatives. More emphasis is being given to the needs of persons in the support networks of families with disabled or chronically ill members. This interest is growing because of the recognized benefits of helping families build and maintain support systems.

For example, some states are starting Grandparent to Grandparent programs. These support groups bring grandparents together to share their strategies and discuss their concerns about helping their children and grandchildren. An experienced grandparent may offer guidance to an inexperienced grandparent. Think how much the grandmother mentioned earlier would have appreciated having someone else to talk to about her fears and concerns.

Friends and relatives are not the only ones who need more information. Lack of information seems to be a particular problem for brothers and sisters of disabled and chronically ill children and adults. The disability and illness have many implications for siblings. For example, some families expect a brother or sister to help take care of the person with a disability or chronic illness. Other siblings must contend with a variety of feelings, such as jealousy, fear, guilt, and resentment. They may feel that there is less money for some of their needs, for example, when a sibling with chronic illness has very high medical costs. Or they may feel uncomfortable inviting friends into their home because they feel embarrassed or they don't know how to answer questions about chronic illness or disability.

Siblings are often given future responsibility for their brother or sister. Siblings are initially part of the immediate family, but as they leave home, marry, and develop their own families, they also become part of the extended network for the young adult with a disability or chronic illness. In one study that interviewed 24 parents of young adults with mental retardation, two-thirds of these parents said it will be the responsibility of their other children to take over when they die. One mother said:

> I talk to my other children about what to expect of Walter. My oldest daughter is very aware that if something happens to me she would be responsible.

Many siblings worry about future responsibility; they are not sure what their role will be and whether they can do the job. Will they have enough money? Will they have enough energy? How will their spouse feel about assuming this responsibility? What about the needs of their own family? One sibling of a woman with mental retardation shared:

> I had just assumed that I would take Faye into my home when mother died. But when I had her for those 3 months (while our elderly mother was ill), I realized I just couldn't do it . . . . I'm not temperamentally suited to it . . . . But I can't put her in a nursing home, I will not do that—I don't know what I'm going to do.

Families can help each other, as well as their social support network, by providing them with information. Sharing information, talking together about plans, and helping people understand the needs surrounding the disability or chronic illness are vital. There are resources to help with this task. In the resource section of this book are the names or sources of several books for siblings, grandparents, aunts, uncles and cousins who would like more information about disability or chronic illness.

Families could also consider asking a relative or a friend to join them when they are working with professionals. If the grandmother who was afraid of hurting her step-granddaughter could be invited along the next time the child's mother meets with a physical therapist, she could learn some basic positioning techniques to help herself feel more comfortable. If the sibling who doesn't know how her sister can be cared for could talk to the staff at her sister's sheltered workshop, she could learn about alternative living opportunities in her community. Maybe there is a group home nearby, or perhaps her sister could live semi-independently with a home care assistant.

If a family is actively involved in their church or synagogue, perhaps they would like information to be available to their clergy and congregation. Although for many families their religious group is the center of social support, many clergy and church and synagogue members have limited knowledge or skills about how to include persons with disability or chronic illness. One father of a severely disabled daughter said:

> Clergy don't have any background with mentally retarded persons. They aren't trained in this area. I wouldn't talk to a fireman, a policeman or a postman about my daughter. Likewise, I wouldn't talk to clergy.

More and more churches and synagogues are working toward more fully including chronically ill and disabled persons and their families in the congregations. Many are conducting awareness training to dispel many of the myths and stereotypes associated with persons who have disability or chronic illness. The American Lutheran Church, one of many religious denominations developing a relationship with persons having disability, has stated the three goals of its ministry as follows:

1. To encourage congregations to eliminate architectural and communication barriers to full participation
2. To work toward eliminating attitudinal barriers that prevent participation of people with disability in the life of the church
3. To encourage advocacy with people with a disability in order to promote services by the church and to affect community change

For many families, their place of worship and its congregation are the focal point of their social support network. In many rural communities the church or synagogue is where the community picnics, clothing is exchanged, and child care services originate.

Providing information about disability to clergy can not only help build social support for families with disabled members but it can also help clergy counsel parents and other family members. When disability enters a family there are often very difficult spiritual questions that arise. How can a God who is good cause this to happen? Is God punishing me for something? Why has God placed this challenge on me? Religious leaders with information about disability are better able to help families with their spiritual interpretations.

Reciprocity

What does reciprocity mean, and why is it so important for building and maintaining social support? Reciprocity means mutual exchange—to give as well as to get. You have probably heard the saying that, to have a friend, you have to be a friend. This is very true in building and maintaining social support.

Imagine that your daughter who has a hearing impairment needs a ride to a summer camp program while your car is being repaired. You know that your neighbor is going on vacation in a couple of weeks and is looking for someone to take in her mail and feed her cats. You could ask your neighbor to provide a ride and also offer to help her out while she is on vacation.

Or suppose the elderly woman down the street seems isolated and lonely since her husband passed away. You know that she would like some visitors, as well as some help with simple chores. You also know that your son with a disability needs a greater variety of social experiences, as well as practice in following through on job tasks. You could discuss with both of them the possibility of his stopping by once a week to empty the trash or carry things to and from the basement.

Recognizing Strengths

Often, friends, relatives, and neighbors think of the problems of a person with a disability or chronic illness without focusing on their strengths. Families can help build and maintain their social support system by helping others recognize the strengths and positive contributions of their family member who has a disability or chronic illness.

Some of the positive contributions that have been identified by others include:

—He has helped me not to take life so seriously.
—She has taught me to be more accepting of differences in people.
—He has taught me that death is part of life.
—She has taught me to take people as they are and to let each person reach his or her own potential.
—She is simply a wonderful person—disability or no disability.

These examples relate more to personal than practical strengths. The more practical strengths can be harder to identify in some situatons, but they are also present. For example, one rural family identified an important strength of their daughter with mental retardation as shared by a sibling:

> You know she can just sit for hours and shuck peas or pick berries and she likes to do it!

For a rural family that depends a lot on gardening for their food supply, this is a very positive contribution that the young woman makes to her family and could make to her social support system as well.

Before a family can help others in their social support network recognize the strengths and positive contributions of the disabled family members, they must be able to recognize these strengths themselves. As part of tapping your own wellspring, think about the positive impacts that a disability or chronic illness has had in your family. What are some ways that those positive contributions can be shared with others?

CHAPTER

4

Who Can Help?

Finding and Using Professional Support

Appropriate professional services can be very necessary and, at times, essential for helping you meet the needs of your family. Many times, you have very realistic concerns and needs that can be addressed by seeking out and using appropriate professionals. There are a range of available professional services that family members need to become familiar with and learn how to gain access to over the years. The range of services include education, medicine, independent living, social work, mental health, law, employment, housing, and recreation. Families with disabled or chronically ill members often come into contact with one or more of these professionals and service agencies. In fact, people we have interviewed often express their confusion or frustration as they try to choose services and then interact with the professionals who want to serve them. This chapter is designed to help you locate professional support and use it most effectively.

Professional support, just like social support, can provide material, emotional, and informational support to your family, as well as to the person with a disability or chronic illness. The types of professional help needed by disabled or chronically ill persons and their families change over time. Awareness of these anticipated changes, however, can help you and your family plan ahead for the type and extent of services that you will need.

The following examples of the professional support that families require at different times illustrate the diverse and changing needs of families. For the mother of a 5-year-old getting ready to start kindergarten, the main concern was obtaining needed service through the school system. She said:

> One thing that still concerns me is that occupational therapy has been drastically overlooked in Sally's life. If she's ever going to learn how to take care of herself—get herself in and out of a wheelchair and things like that—she's going to have to have someone to work directly with her every day to teach her how. We specified that in her IEP [individualized education program], but I know the public schools do not have the staff to provide this . . . . So that's one thing I'll really have to follow up on.

Another mother of a 15-year-old son was most concerned about finding and securing available recreational opportunities for her son. She said:

> My greatest need right now is to see Walter involved in athletic activities. He doesn't get much opportunity and he really likes that sort of thing. I know it would improve his self-confidence. But we live in a rural area and transportation is a real problem for us.

A father of a 25-year-old son said his greatest formal support need at this time in his son's life was for residential services.

> There is a great need for housing for the physically disabled. There comes a time when every child needs to cut the apron strings, but there is little barrier-free housing available across the country. More housing is needed, especially for my son.

The wife of a 54-year-old man who has been disabled by a head injury is seeking personal care support:

> What I really need is a personal care attendant to take care of Adam. He's too heavy for me to lift and bathe and dress. He wouldn't have to stay in bed all day if someone could come in and help twice a day.

Finally, the daughter of an 80-year-old woman with cancer felt her mother's greatest need was for social activities:

The Visiting Nurses Association comes in every day to help Mom out with her bathing and meals, and that's nice. But I'd also like to see her involved in some sort of social program. Something where they come and get her and take her where she'll be around other people. She needs to be more active than she is now.

These families are seeking different types of professional help at five different stages of life. The diagram in Figure 1 graphically illustrates how professional support needs change over the lifetime of a person with a disability or chronic illness. The six pie charts represent six different stages of the life cycle. Each professional service has a different-sized piece of pie at different life stages. The services at different life cycle stages also vary, depending on the type of disability or chronic illness. For example, for a degenerative chronic illness, the medical support needs would probably increase over the life cycle. For a mental illness, mental health services would need to be added at a later point.

One of the keys to the effective use of professional support is thinking ahead to the types of support you will need in the future. Finding services, going through the application process, or getting on the waiting list all take time.

As you look at the charts in the figure, think of the illness or disability within your own family. What types of services would you add or delete? What types of services will you need next year? Five years from now? Future planning can help you get a head start on locating and examining the services you will need.

ROADBLOCKS TO DEVELOPING FORMAL SUPPORT

You may encounter many roadblocks in obtaining professional and community services for yourself or your disabled or chronically ill family member throughout the lifespan. As you read the following discussion about these roadblocks, think about some of the problems your family has already encountered. After you have identified your own family roadblocks, we suggest some ways that those roadblocks can be addressed to enable you to build and maintain professional support to help with your family needs.

Lack of Coordinated Services

The services required by a family with a disabled family member are numerous, and they are offered by a wide variety of professionals and

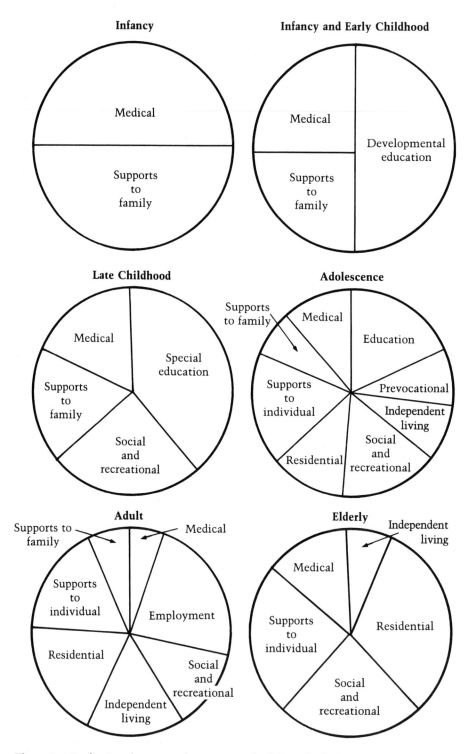

Figure 1. Professional support changes over the life cycle. [Adapted from Murphy, A. (1983). Community services and resources within the family. In J. A. Mulick & S. M. Pueschel (eds.), *Parent-professional partnership in developmental disability services.* Cambridge, MA: Academic Guild.]

agencies. Ideally, a family would only have to go to one place to coordinate all those services. Unfortunately, very few communities offer such a coordinating service. To make coordination even more difficult, there is often limited communication among such programs as education, health, mental health, and various social services. One agency often doesn't know what the other is doing. There can be several service providers in the same town who are unaware of the services offered by each other. To address this problem, some communities are currently working toward interagency coordination, an effort to link together services within a community.

The service delivery system can be thought of as a bureaucratic maze, and negotiating that maze is a large task for families. One father of a 26-year-old daughter with cerebral palsy, when asked what his greatest need was, responded:

> I would like some central source of information, like a *Who's Who* in a library—a place to get information on what's happening, what's available, where is the money? The biggest problem is keeping up with what is available. And how to get it.

In a few communities, there are central sources of information and referral. An information and referral center can help families know what is available, but lack of coordination between service agencies can still exist. Many professional agencies are working toward coordination of services, but they have a long way to go.

Cost

A major roadblock for many families to using formal support and services is financial cost. One mother of a 4-year-old physically disabled daughter stated her greatest need as:

> Money! Do you have a million dollars? I don't. Money is so important to the future security of my daughter. Financial needs are our greatest concern—to be able to cover expenses yearly and monthly.

The father of a 26-year-old son who has spina bifida said the most stressful experience for his family was:

> Finding finances. I don't know where the money is going to come from. We've had to have help over the years. I quit counting when Ron's hospital bills topped $600,000.

Some services, such as public education and community recreation programs, are publicly funded and free to families. However, others, such as medical or mental health services, have either firmly set fees or use a sliding fee scale. If a service that you need costs more money than you have, that's a difficult roadblock to overcome. Yet, you have several options. After searching, you might locate another agency to finance the service or offer the service free. Some agencies might provide information on sources of aid to help you attain needed services. As we noted in Chapter 3, using social support requires you to provide some kind of help in return to the friends and neighbors who help you. Building social support requires an investment of time and energy. But when finances are limited, an investment of time and energy in social support may be an alternative to professional support.

Planning for the financial security of the disabled person is a concern that many families share. How to set up a will? How to do estate planning? How to have access to such governmental benefit programs as Social Security Disability Income (SSDI) or Supplemental Security Income (SSI)? Because the discussion of these issues is beyond the scope of this book, we have included a list of publications providing information on financial planning in the resource section.

Attitudes of Professionals

The organized efforts of helping professionals are aimed at providing support to persons with a disability or chronic illness and their families. Although these interactions are meant to be supportive, the history of professional–family relationships has not always been positive.

Professionals vary greatly in their attitudes toward persons with disabilities or chronic illness and their families. There are many different perspectives that professionals bring to their work. Some professionals are taught that their job is to cure a disease, impart knowledge, or rehabilitate persons so that they can fully function on a job or at home. They may attack the problem without regard for the emotional needs of the individuals involved. When the problem doesn't completely go away, as is the case with disabilities or chronic illness, these professionals may not be able to avoid feeling that they have somehow failed. Unfortunately, the all-too-human reaction of some of these professionals is to dismiss the individual and his or her family. This is sometimes the unconscious motivation of professionals who encourage institutionalization without considering other options. As one mother of a young mentally retarded son said:

> At birth the doctor said to put him in an institution, he would never be more than a vegetable. We were a new thing for professionals, especially doctors. In those years all children were placed in institutions. But we accepted the challenge and it has been exciting.

The wife of a man with a severe disability shared:

> I have seen two physicians in 11 years. That's my only contact with professionals. At the time of the accident a medical doctor said, "Put him in a home or institution right away. That would be best for your family." Now, 11 years later, another doctor advises to place him in a home for awhile to relieve the pressure and physical care needs.

Interviews with family members provide evidence that, rather than being a source of support to families, some professionals are a source of additional stress. There are, however, many professionals who focus on the strengths of families and individuals and who do provide support. They believe in developing the unique potential of each individual. Many people have told us about professionals who listened, provided needed information, and helped families to cope. One mother of a young son with asthma said:

> I have had a lot of professionals who have hung in there with us and helped me with Mark. We have been blessed with good professionals to work with. In general, they have been thoughtful, sensitive, and helpful.

The husband of a woman with muscular dystrophy talked about his wife's doctor:

> Shauna's doctor has been so important to me because he really cares. He has given good advice and is always supportive of her. I feel like she or I can call him at any time.

Just as in any field, there are helpful professionals and there are unhelpful professionals in the field of disability and chronic illness. It is very disheartening to encounter the unhelpful ones. When seeking out professionals to help meet your family needs, don't waste time on those who have negative attitudes. There are other professionals available who believe in the strengths and potential of all your family members. Exercise 4A may be useful to you; think of professionals who have been helpful to you, and list the things that made the experience helpful. Think also of professionals who were unhelpful, and list how you could have handled the interaction differently. Thinking about these issues may assist you in choosing positive professionals and working with them more efficiently.

Exercise 4A

1. Think of a professional who has been particularly helpful to you. List some of the things that made the experience successful for you.

2. Think of a professional who was particularly *unhelpful* to you. List what was unhelpful about him or her. In retrospect, is there some way you could have handled the interaction differently?

Jargon

Another roadblock you may have encountered in building and using formal support is the use of jargon. Jargon is the specialized language professionals use primarily to talk to each other and secondarily to talk to you as the receiver of services. As the daughter of a woman with Alzheimer's disease told us:

> I don't know of any professionals I can talk to. Let me know if there are any that know anything. If there was someone we could communicate with, we would. But there aren't any professionals in gerontology who can talk.

In any profession there are a certain number of phrases, initials, and language shortcuts that help professionals work more efficiently. The fields of disability and chronic illness have their own share of jargon. Here are a few examples of initials that professionals may use:

HHS—Health and Human Services
SRS—Social Rehabilitation Services
SSI—Supplemental Security Income
SSDI—Social Security Disability Insurance
MR—Mental retardation
MS—Muscular dystrophy
CP—Cerebral palsy
VR—Vocational rehabilitation
LRE—Least restrictive environment
MI—Mental illness
IEP—Individualized education program
IPP—Individualized program plan

Professionals in the fields of disability and chronic illness use many abbreviations and technical terms. Don't be afraid to ask professionals to tell you in simple language what they are talking about. Jargon only keeps a distance in communication between professionals and family members. Confronting some professionals may threaten their self-esteem. But they not only owe simple language to you, they also owe it to themselves. Professionals have a responsibility to talk to anyone, particularly the people they serve, in a language that is clear, concise, and understandable.

Stigma

In Chapter 3 we noted that some families may avoid building a support network because they fear the possibility of stigma or social rejection. This is equally true of professional support. A predominant social attitude held by many people in society, including some professionals, is that those people who are different are somehow inferior to those who are not. Family members of the person who is disabled or chronically ill are also viewed as different or as part of the problem.

This social stigma is beginning to change in our society. Persons with disability and chronic illness are becoming a more visible and vocal minority. They are speaking up for their own rights. More and more, they are being looked on as people who are valuable, equal, contributing members of society. Still, some professionals practicing today might not yet have lost some of the earlier views about disability or chronic illness. The fear of confronting professionals who will stigmatize you is real, particularly if you are poor, a member of a minority, or have less assertive communication skills.

Stigma is present in our society, and you will encounter it. But remember, there are professionals who will focus on your strengths, regard you as an equal, respect and admire you, and listen to your needs. Remember to speak up for your rights. For example, you may get faster service in the doctor's office if you are able to say, "I have been waiting 45 minutes for my appointment; I have many other important things to do today, so I would appreciate it if you would tell the doctor to see me as soon as possible." For more information on using direct and assertive communication skills, read the several books on this topic listed in the resource section.

Time and Energy

One of the biggest roadblocks is the time and energy needed to acquire and use professional support. It takes a lot of time and energy to locate services, make phone calls, drive to appointments, review records, attend conferences, fill out forms, and visit programs. Time is needed to obtain, use, evaluate, monitor, and change every service.

Each family has a different amount of time and energy it can invest in using professional support. There are only 24 hours in a day, and in this finite amount of time, your needs and the needs of everyone else in the family must be met. Family members sometimes forget that their own personal needs are as legitimate as the person's needs with the disability or chronic illness. One father who is the single parent of a son with leukemia said:

> At certain times many demands are made of me, like transportation to therapy sessions. I have to adjust my whole life to fit his. This is very difficult to do and work at the same time. There's a lack of freedom from this. I feel like I never have time to do anything. But I guess it teaches me to be organized.

The point here is that the time and energy it takes to get and use professional services must be measured against the time and energy your family has for the other things that are also important.

Lack of Service

Probably one of the biggest roadblocks to using professional support is that sometimes it doesn't exist. Especially in rural areas, even if you had the money, time, and energy, there may be few services to use. One elderly mother of an adult who is mentally retarded said:

One home is too high-functioning; another one is too low. I have looked and looked. She will probably have to quit her job and move in with her brother when I die. She will probably just sit there because the city he lives in doesn't have anything to offer.

Even when services are available, there are often very long waiting lists to get them. This is why, as we noted earlier, it is important to plan ahead and begin looking for services *before* you need them. Or you might be able to fill some needs by relying on your social support network. As you read Part II, "Problem Solving," think about creative ways to meet your needs when services are lacking. Exercise 4B may help you identify your roadblocks to using professional support, as well as ways to overcome those roadblocks.

BUILDING AND MAINTAINING PROFESSIONAL SUPPORT

Building and maintaining formal support can be hindered by many roadblocks, but many of them can be overcome. The following four methods can help you bypass those roadblocks.

1. *Case management*—ways to help you be the manager of your own situation
2. *Positive attitude*—attitudes that can help you deal more effectively with professionals
3. *Support groups*—peer support and information about having access to formal support
4. *Advocates*—who they are and how to use them

Case Management

One way to help overcome many of the roadblocks to using professional support is to take over the job of case manager. This means keeping your own records and securing and coordinating your own services. It can be a big task. As one professional describes it:

> At any point in time a severely handicapped person may be receiving services from 4–6 different agencies and may be in contact with 15–20 different professionals. With each of these different agencies and each of these highly specialized professionals assuming its own role, the attainment of continuity, coordination, and consistency of services can be a problem of considerable magnitude. It is the parents and the family, then,

---

Exercise 4B

1. List the roadblocks you have experienced in using professional support. We have listed a few, but include any others your family has encountered.

2. Select one roadblock and list possible ways to overcome that roadblock. Discuss your ideas with other family members.

---

who are left with the primary responsibility of creating order out of what may seem to be a chaotic situation (Lyons & Preis, 1983, p. 213).

Many times, persons with disability or chronic illness or their family members don't have the skills to be their own case managers. However, some service programs, such as independent living resource centers, are increasingly recognizing that the key to ensuring services to persons with disabilities or chronic illness and their families is to teach them these skills. Professionals and service programs come and go. You and your family are the most dependable resource over your lifetime.

People who can be articulate about exactly what they want, what services they have had in the past, and what goals and objectives they are working toward are more likely to receive better services on a long-term basis. When meeting with professionals, it is very important to state your own choices for services and goals. When persons with a disability or chronic illness are very young, the parents might have to interpret what their children's choices and preferences would be. As these persons grow older, they may take greater responsibility for stating their own needs and choices commensurate with their ability. This responsibility would have to be determined on an individual basis, however, because some illnesses, such as Alzheimer's disease, may require a greater need for support as the person gets older.

Table 4.1 offers some helpful tips about locating and using professional services.

Table 4.1. Tips to use in locating professional support

Method	Suggestion
The telephone is a good place to start.	Give your name, and ask for the appropriate person or state your reason for calling. If the person to whom you wish to speak is not available, leave your name, phone number and a message. Find out approximately when your call will be returned.
A letter often becomes a necessary form of communication, particularly when a telephone call has not worked.	State your need and the reason you are writing. Be brief and to the point. Address the proper person if you know his or her name. Keep a carbon copy of the letter for your files.
Recordkeeping helps you to stay organized and develop confidence as a case manager.	Get copies of school, medical, and other important records. Keep a list of whom you have contacted, when, and the outcome. Prepare a standard background sheet that includes health and medical history, and history of contacts with other service providers. This sheet may be given to new professionals, avoiding repetition and saving you time.

Adapted from Rubin and Quinn-Curran (1983, p. 78).

Positive Attitude

What is an attitude? It is the state of mind with which you approach a situation. A positive attitude toward working with professionals greatly affects how successful you are in achieving your goals. A positive attitude can make problems easier to handle, goals more attainable, mistakes less disastrous, and the future more exciting.

It is helpful not to be too critical of professionals. They are often painfully aware of their own limitations—not enough staff to go around, not enough money to meet everyone's needs, too little knowledge about what to do. Try to give them credit for doing their best, even when it isn't enough. One mother of a young son with mental retardation explained her strategy for working with professionals.

> Mark's pediatrician has been most helpful to me over the years. It's all in your approach. If you are willing to meet people half-way, they will be cooperative.

Often, professionals only hear from family members when there are complaints or problems. Just like everyone else, they need to hear about the good things they do. Dealing with professionals in a positive, assertive, and considerate manner can be essential to attaining the help you need.

Support Groups

As we noted in Chapter 3, support groups can help you locate and use professional support. They can also help meet a variety of needs, such as providing information on the following: legal rights, who are helpful professionals, how to avoid redtape, which programs are good, or how to plan for the future.

Many parents have reported valuable emotional support and information from support groups. One mother of a preschool daughter with spina bifida said:

> Talking to the other parents is great—it helps to share with people. It's only through talking to other parents that you find out what doctor prescribes medication or who will tell you more than just not to worry. I have learned more about services by talking to parents than any professional.

Support groups need not only be for parents or, most usually, only for mothers. Communities are beginning to organize support groups for fathers, siblings, grandparents, spouses, and many others whose lives are touched by disability or chronic illness. Of particular note are the increasing number of self-advocacy groups that bring people with disability or chronic illness together to share their own experiences and to advocate for services. Particular groups vary greatly in their goals and the amount of commitment expected from members. Groups sometimes exist to accomplish a specific task, such as building a group home. Although most support groups are helpful, some support groups could be depressive or disempowering. Choose your groups wisely, and be prepared that a certain group might not meet your needs.

For the addresses of some local support groups and for more information, refer to the "Resources" appendix at the back of the book for a listing of many national organizations. These organizations can help you locate support groups in your area.

Advocacy

Because family members are the most consistent individuals in your life, they can often be your best advocates. Each family, however, varies in the amount of time, energy, knowledge, and finances available to take on this role. One mother who was describing her struggle to find housing and attendant care services said:

> Advocates are needed who could help families with this work. So much energy is spent on getting services and parents don't always know where to go.

Many formal agencies, schools included, often make committed and active effort toward providing the most appropriate service for an individual with a disability or chronic illness. But their services are often hard to find and use. Other agencies or programs may just try to fit individuals in whether it is appropriate or not.

If families need or want help in securing appropriate services, they can enlist the support of an advocate. An advocate is someone who assists the individual in acquiring appropriate services. This person can be a friend, relative, or someone professionally skilled at being an advocate. Organizations exist to provide help to people with disabilities or chronic illness and their families as they advocate for their legal rights or try to gain access to services. Many community independent living centers have a specialist who can help advocate for services or benefits. For people with developmental disabilities, every state has a federally sponsored protection and advocacy agency that might be helpful. Consult a state directory or ask a professional how you can contact the protection and advocacy agency in your state. Their services are free of charge.

In addition, family members with a disability or chronic illness should be encouraged to be an advocate for themselves. Beginning at an early age, they could be encouraged to attend planning meetings and actively participate in setting goals.

PUTTING IT ALL TOGETHER

Even in areas where few services exist, every family with a disabled or chronically ill member comes into at least some contact with professionals. Services are available to provide you with material, emotional, and informational support. The trick is that you must first locate services and then work successfully with the professionals in these agencies. You can accomplish these tasks by piecing together information from other families and people you meet, as well as from educators, rehabilitation counselors, doctors, psychologists, and other professionals you already know. The "Resources" appendix in this book is another place to start.

When you put together the information from both Chapters 3 and 4, you might begin to realize that you have an impressive array of resources at your disposal. The next step is deciding just how to put those resources to work. To do this, you should have a full understanding of the various needs of all your family members.

CHAPTER

5

Everybody Has Needs

As we discussed in Chapter 1, families are extremely busy. Most of us easily identify with the hustle-bustle of family life. Whether family life involves the family with young children, the single parent with an adolescent, the newly married couple, an elderly couple whose children have grown and gone, or a huge and close extended family network, families form the hub of activity and intimacy in our complex and diverse lives. What is the purpose of all this activity?

By and large, families exist to meet the individual and collective needs of their members. All of us have a wide range of economic, physical, and emotional needs. We tend to think of a need as something we don't have, but we also have needs that we are fairly satisfied are being fulfilled. Some of us have many unmet needs; others have only a few. Whether they are met or unmet, however, individual needs are usually addressed in the context of family living.

Having a member with a disability accentuates some needs and decreases others. As one mother said in regard to her physically disabled daughter:

> Having other children, we had our own control group. When you don't have a comparison, everything looms big. Raising kids is a hassle! Paula takes time, but I never had to be a Brownie leader, or take her to piano lessons, or enforce a curfew. Paula is the least of the problems after having raised three teenagers in the decade of the 1970s.

In order to help families function successfully, it is useful to look at the many varied needs that families have, paying special attention to both the positive and negative impacts that a family member with a disability or illness may have on those needs.

Over the last 100 years, we have gradually turned over many of the need-fulfilling functions of the family to outside social groups. Schools educate our children; clothing and food are frequently ready-made and purchased outside the home; even recreational and cultural experiences are often provided by the community where they once were provided by the family (for example, we go to ball games or watch TV, rather than participate in "group sings" around the piano). Perhaps the growing number of people living alone is testimony to this trend. However, even people living alone are still attached to family (or families). Whether or not the family actually performs the tasks involved in serving individual needs, the family is still the context within which most of us live and address our needs. Families are the orchestrators of the resources that serve, or try to serve, their members' needs.

Family members are interdependent in that they rely on each other to fulfill many essential needs. A hearing-impaired man, married to a woman who also has a hearing impairment, told us:

> There was a time that I wanted to pride myself on being independent. But God didn't create us to be on our own. I think we're meant out of necessity to be interdependent. I don't think our ultimate goal is complete and total "independence."

Ultimately, the pay-off from such cooperation of energy and resources is increased independence to live one's life to its fullest. Thus, family members acquire independence through the very interdependence that enables them to meet their needs.

What exactly are these needs that families try to address? Although many ideas may immediately cross your mind, it may be helpful to categorize these ideas into eight basic areas of family needs. Family needs include: 1) economic, 2) health and security, 3) physical caretaking, 4) social, 5) recreational, 6) affectional, 7) self-definitional, and 8) educational requirements. Some of these needs may immediately impress you as being more important than others, as well they should. Every family places varying degrees of emphasis on different needs, some valuing recreation and economics to a greater degree and others affection or education. Similarly, some of these may strike you as unimportant because there may be more pressing needs that are going unmet in your family. For example, families for whom finances are a constant source of distress may not have the time, resources, or even an interest, in meeting recreational needs. It is also important to remember that needs change over time. The needs that are most important to a family with infants or preschoolers are probably not the same ones that receive attention in a family with adolescents or young adults. Before exploring the special met and unmet needs in your own family and how they change, we first describe the eight areas of needs in more detail.

THE EIGHT BASIC FAMILY NEEDS

Economic

As you well know, economic survival is an unavoidable reality in today's society. In order to meet this need, family members engage in a number of activities geared toward attaining and allocating finances. For example, family members work, manage the budget, and decide how the money will be spent. The presence of a member with a disability or illness often affects both the amount of money a family needs, as well as the amount it is able to produce. Even in families with insurance, medical bills can be devastating. Motorized wheelchairs, lift vans, ramps for stairs, and grab-bars for bathrooms are expenses to be faced by families with a disabled member. Medicine, home-nursing care, and specialized diets for someone with a chronic illness can be very expensive. Even babysitters are more expensive for a child with special needs. The list of costs associated with disabilities and illnesses goes on and on. Only a few of the very wealthiest families are unaffected.

At the same time that costs increase, the family's ability to make money may be reduced. Depending on the special need, earning capacity may be reduced for the disabled or chronically ill person. In addition, one or more members of the family may make job sacrifices, either to care for the disabled or ill person or to have access to resources. One man with a physical disability told us:

> My dad turned down a promotional opportunity in another city because the school system did not have mainstreaming. He believed I should be in

a regular school. He was very upfront about why he turned down the promotion, and I felt badly about it. It wasn't a really bad guilt trip, but those feelings were there.

Many families face difficulties in meeting the economic needs of their members. Although economic difficulties are not unique to families with disabled or chronically ill members, you may at times encounter more financial burdens than do other families. The specific disability or illness in your family may result in more or less expenses than do others, or your family may have greater or fewer resources to cope with the costs. We have no magical suggestions for doing away with financial problems. Many of us, however, could manage better with the resources we have. Included in the resource section of this book are some books on basic money management techniques that you and your family may find helpful.

Health and Security

The health and security needs of a family are central to its sense of well-being. Family members strive individually and collectively to maintain good health—perhaps by eating right, getting enough rest, exercising, and seeing a physician on a regular basis. Similarly, the family functions to meet members' needs for security, to feel that they are safe and wanted in a comfortable and dependable atmosphere. Thus, health and security are important needs to which the family attends in the course of daily life.

Having a member with a disability or illness in the family can affect these needs. For example, health needs may become the #1 priority in a family that consistently deals with physical or mental health problems in one of its members. The daughter of a woman with Alzheimer's disease said:

> When we brought Mother home, the hospital staff told us that she had only about a year to live. That was hard! For a long time after that, every time she sneezed or got sick we panicked.

Similarly, attitudes toward health care workers can be either positively or negatively influenced by family members' interactions with such professionals as physicians, psychologists, and physical therapists. These attitudes can influence family members' desire to seek out these services and attend to these needs.

The security needs of a family can also be affected by lack of knowledge about what the future holds. For example, it may be difficult to feel secure and settled if plans have not been made for the future adult care of a member with a disability. Similarly, the unpredictable nature of some illnesses may make insecurity an unavoidable part of life for some families, to be dealt with as best as possible. The mother of a son with severe behavior problems described her family situation:

> As much as we value security, it is a fragile condition in our home. We never know from one day to the next, even from one hour to the next, whether peace or aggression will reign. We can think everything is calm, and the next minute Larry can explode with intense outbursts of hitting and choking. Even when he is calm, we can never be caught with our guard down. We long for the security of what home should provide, but we learn to live with insecurity. Nothing is more important to us than overcoming this family problem so that home will be a safe place.

Health and security are needs to which families with members having special needs are often particularly attuned. Each family must address these needs based on its own unique situation.

Physical

Physical needs refer to the day-to-day requirements of living: cooking, laundry, cleaning, shopping, and so forth. Some persons with special needs may need extra help with such needs as dressing, bathing, and eating. Chronic illnesses may require nursing care or put special constraints on the performance of routine chores. For example, because a person with diabetes must eat meals at more or less regular times a fixed schedule for meal preparation and eating may be imposed on a family that values mealtimes together. One group of parents reported that the physical caretaking of a child with a disability took an average of 2 hours per day. Yet, although the time and energy involved in fulfilling physical needs may be considerable, it may actually take more time and energy to help enable a person with a disability to care for him or herself. One sibling said:

> My brother was always pampered by Mom, and I always thought she should allow him to do more for himself. But when he came to live with me for a year, I realized I was not helping his independence either. I learned it was easier and quicker to do things for him than to let him do for himself.

Although physical needs may be demanding of certain family members' resources, alternatives that can distribute this responsibility to other family members, persons in the community, or persons with a disability themselves often exist. It may take more time and energy to set up these alternatives initially, but in the long run, doing so could help the person with a disability acquire more independence. In turn, this may help the family meet the continuing physical needs of all members.

Recreation

The family serves an important role in fulfilling family members' needs to relax, enjoy, and be themselves. We all need a break every now and then from daily responsibilities, and the family household can provide an undemanding atmosphere for enjoying rest and recreation.

The family's ability to engage in recreational activities can be reduced by a member with special needs. As with other needs, the impact of a disability or illness on recreational options is largely dependent on its type and level of severity. Stress can often result from trying to participate in nonaccessible recreational options.

Taking a break from chronic responsibilities can be a form of recreation in itself for family care providers. The husband of a woman with osteogenesis imperfecta said:

> I used to turn down chances to go places with my friends and have fun, but then I found myself starting to resent Carol. I would mope around the house feeling sorry for myself. Carol finally convinced me to go ahead and take off once in awhile. I now feel that's what has saved our relationship.

Family members who choose to make time for rest and relaxation away from their disabled or chronically ill family member should strive to keep guilt from creeping into their enjoyment. Everyone has needs for recreation, and the needs of each member in the family are equally important.

One mother, a single parent of a 5-year-old with mental retardation shared with us her delight that, for the first time in 5 years she had taken time just for herself, to go do just what she wanted to do. She exclaimed:

> I'm doing something for the development of my mental health—all by myself. For the first time since Lisa's birth, I'm doing something just for me without feeling quilty.

Thus, spending time away from day-to-day pressures is a need that rejuvenates us and makes life more enjoyable. For the individual who is disabled or ill, more and more recreational opportunities are being made available within communities. The resource section of this book provides information on a variety of recreational alternatives.

Socialization

Families are the base from which people learn how to interact with one another. Children first learn how to interact with siblings and parents and then graduallly branch out from this social foundation to the outside world. Thus, the family can fulfill the crucial need of preparing us for social relationships, on both an informal and an intimate level.

A family member with a special need often has an impact on socialization. For example, it can sometimes be difficult to provide persons with severe and multiple disabilities opportunities to interact with nondisabled people, yet these experiences can be valuable for all concerned. For many families, going out in public and dealing with stares from strangers and questions from friends seems to be a source of stress. Siblings often experience embarrassment in social situations. One sister with an older brother who is mentally retarded commented:

> When we go to the movies or to church, Al talks out and everyone turns around to look. I know what they're thinking. They think he's "dumb" and then they look at me and think I'm "dumb" too.

Parents and spouses may feel angry about staring strangers and insensitive neighbors. Others may feel jealous of the opportunities that most people can enjoy that their own loved ones cannot. As the wife of a man with paraplegia said:

> Yesterday at work the men in my office were bragging about the softball game they'd won the other day. I kept thinking that Pete would love terribly to play softball, not only because of the fun of it, but because of this special camaraderie and attention all these men enjoyed. I wanted to tell them to quit their bragging, already!

Thus, families can sometimes feel left out of the social mainstream or even isolate themselves from others because of their anger, resentment, and embarrassment.

However, the experience of having a family member with a special need can also prove extremely rewarding in terms of social relationships. Family members learn to benefit from the helping hands of individuals both in and outside the family, as well as how to give of themselves. As the sister of a woman with cancer said:

> Your attitudes toward people end up being extremely good. Every time we needed someone's time they were so giving—all these people really helped us out.

Similarly, the person with a disability or illness may demonstrate a special attitude towards others that may be inspirational to the whole family. As one mother of a son with mental retardation observed:

> Josh does have a positive expectation to be accepted. He loves to shake hands with whomever he meets, and he expects everyone to like him. I think that is a *very neat* characteristic. Even though Josh has given very few clues of feeling rejected, there is certainly something that lights up in him when he is around people whom he knows accept him and love him. Greater than Josh's need to be in his familiar surroundings is his need to be with the people he loves. That says a lot about the quality of Josh's love. It is abiding, constant, and unwavering. His need is to have that same quality of love reciprocated from other people.

One woman with muscular dystrophy became a source of inspiration and courage for her entire inner-city neighborhood:

> Everybody loved Aunt Cornelia. Some of us would get mad about how her life turned out—she worked hard all her life and now this was her reward. But she never complained. She always loved company, always wanted to hear how the young ones were getting on in school, always listened to everybody's troubles and had a good word to say to this one or that. Sometimes I still say to myself, when I hit a rough spot—if Aunt Cornelia could handle all she did and still come away smiling, why, for sure I ought to be able to handle this.

Self-Definition

We all have a need to determine who we are and define for ourselves both our role in society and our identity as individuls. Families play a very important role in helping us establish our self-identities. For the person with a special need, some families may have expectations that are too high and some that are too low. Often, families thwart self-expression and development by discounting the disabled or chronically ill member's potential and limiting his or her activity. Or a family may feel a need to overprotect its disabled or ill members. As the mother of a daughter with mental retardation explained:

I was fearful of rape with her. But then our other daughter lived in a bad neighborhood in the city. So with normal children there are risks, and with mentally retarded children there are risks.

In some families, hopes and expectations are not limited. This attitude can enable family members to view the individual as a person first and as someone with a special need second. As one sibling of a brother with four prosthetic limbs put it:

People would ask me what's with your brother. I couldn't relate to the question. I would say something like, "He has a cold" . . . we never saw our brother as any different.

An often-overlooked fact is that a person with a disability or illness can affect the identity of other family members as significantly as they can affect his or hers. For example, siblings sometimes feel guilty about achieving more than a disabled brother or sister or about feeling healthy when a sibling is ill. Likewise, a spouse may restrict his or her freedom in order to avoid emphasizing differences in ability or freedom. Parents sometimes have their identities wholly invested in their disabled or ill child, feeling worthwhile because "God entrusted me with this special child." Adult sons or daughters who must take over responsibility for an aging parent often feel a sense of confusion over the switch of roles, where once they depended on their mother or father for guidance, now they are the "parents." Often, when an individual's self-definition becomes wrapped up in the care of the member with a special need, the family can restrict both itself and the person with a special need from fully developing beyond the singular self-concept of being disabled or ill. The excitement and pride of surpassing such artificial limitations with even the most seemingly minor achievements are illustrated by a 10-year-old girl with a hearing impairment:

Mother and father order for me all the time. I choose what I want to eat and tell them, but I never show the waitress myself. But last year I went with my friend's aunt to McDonald's and I ordered all by myself!

Affection

Although the amounts vary among individuals, everyone needs affection. Often, the family is the major, if not the sole, source of affection for its members. A disabled or chronically ill family member can have both a positive and a negative impact on the family's ability to meet its members' affectional needs. For example, a sense of being different can draw a family closer together and give them a strong sense of belonging to a special unit. A life-threatening or terminal illness can give a family a heightened sense of appreciation and love for one another. Most families are able to identify the benefits of having a special family member with this type of intangible value: "She taught me how to care," "she helped me to appreciate life," or "he taught me to accept people where they are."

A negative impact may also occur in families with members with a disability or illness. For example, if a disproportionate amount of the parents' time is spent caring for a disabled or ill child, the other children may feel neglected and have unmet affectional needs. Parents may withdraw from each other if they blame themselves or each other for their child's illness or disability (e.g., "If only I had insisted she stay home that night"). In adult couples, the sexual needs of one or both partners may be neglected if open communication is not established. Thus, again we see how one person's needs can directly affect another's needs in a family and how important communication is in addressing issues as they arise.

Often, some family members do not understand the intimate and sexual needs of the disabled or chronically ill person. Many parents of sons and daughters with disabilities or illnesses feel that their children's sexual needs do not exist. As one mother of an adolescent son with a disability said:

> He has no needs along this line. I don't see any sexual desires expressed. He asked, "Will I ever get married?" and I said, "No." Besides, it is against the church.

Another mother of a physically disabled young adult was more open about her son's need for affection:

> I told Ron to find some girl at camp that would take him home with her. He laughed, and said, "I'll try, Mom."

The affectional and sexual needs of persons with disabilities and illnesses vary, depending on the individual and the degree and type of disability. Nonetheless, needs for intimacy and sexual expression exist in all persons. The resource section of this book lists several references that can help persons with disabilities and their families better understand and confront these needs.

Education

Particularly in families with children, educational needs are addressed on a frequent basis. In fact, educational needs may not even be consciously considered, but may be naturally met in the course of parent-child and sibling relationships. For example, having books in the home, discussing current events, washing the car, or taking trips to museums all fulfill educational needs.

Families vary greatly in the degree of emphasis they place on education and the importance of developing a vocation. Often, however, this need is overlooked for and by the disabled or ill family member. As one mother remarked:

> Work is not high on Maslow's hierarchy of needs. Survival is most important. Most of all she needs a place to live and be happy and get love. The rest is extra.

Parents might not have expectations that their son or daughter will ever work, so they do not plan for it. Similarly, because of a non-disabled spouse's lowered expectations, a recently disabled spouse might not be expected to carry out responsibilities he or she formerly performed. On the other side of the coin, families can also over-emphasize educational development to the exclusion of meeting other needs. Sondra Diamond (1981), a psychologist who has a physical disability, wrote in reaction to her parent's emphasis on therapeutic training at home:

> Something happens in a parent when relating to his disabled child; he forgets that they're a kid first. I used to think about that a lot when I was a kid. I would be off in a euphoric state, drawing or coloring or cutting out paper dolls, and as often as not the activity would be turned into an occupational therapy session. "You're not holding the scissors right," "Sit up straight so your curvature doesn't get worse." That era was ended when I finally let loose a long and exhaustive tirade. "I'm just a kid! You can't therapize me all the time! I get enough therapy in school every day! I don't think about my handicap all the time like you do!" (p. 30).

It is important to stress the fact that each family emphasizes some needs more than others. In a family placing a low value on recreation, there are likely to be fewer forms of entertainment in the home and fewer excursions outside the home. Families may also serve the needs of some members more than others. For example, a husband and wife may "sacrifice" their need to be alone together in order to care for their children. These variations depend strictly on the individual values and needs of a given family, as no two families are ever alike in terms of how they meet their unique constellation of needs.

How about your own family? Chances are you recognized many of your own needs in our discussion of the eight types of family needs. Exercise 5A is designed to help you clarify what your needs are and how currently satisfied you are that they are being met. Try to get as many people in your family to fill it out, either by making copies of the exercise or by using different colored pens for each person.

Did some of your answers surprise you? No doubt, you see many areas of need that require improvement in the opinion of one or more family members. But before you focus on problems, stop and take pride in the many needs your family *is* meeting. Every "3" or "4" in Column B is a mark of family strength. You should congratulate each other—and yourself—on getting so much done.

No doubt also your family members didn't agree 100% on the importance placed on certain needs or on how satisfied they were. This is as it should be. Just as every family is unique, so is every individual in each family. There are no right or wrong answers in this exercise, and everyone's needs are legitimate. Nor should pinpointing unmet needs be a source of guilt or blame. Rather, we hope you will look at needs you think are important (scores of 3 or 4 in Column A) but still unmet (scores of 1 or 2 in Column B) as goals to strive toward as you begin to build your family strengths.

By now you are probably thinking of many areas of need you would like to address—but how? There are, after all, only 24 hours in a day. The prospect of squeezing in just one more task can feel overwhelming. But there are ways to tackle the problem. It may be that you can recruit some of the people you identified in Chapter 3 to help out. Or you may want to look into some possible help from the professionals or agencies available to you. Before taking a closer look at your people resources, however, we'd like you to consider another strategy that has gained a great deal of popularity in recent years: time management.

GETTING MORE DONE

Time management is an important issue in the business world. Employers sponsor seminars on this subject, and business schools are beginning to discuss effective time management in their curricula. A new book on the topic seems to appear every month or so. There is no reason why effective use of time can't be applied to family life—and indeed, there are several good books and articles available. No doubt

Exercise 5A

Below is a list of needs common to most families, organized within each of the eight basic areas of need. We have left some blanks in each area for you to add any other needs that might be special to your family. First, consider how important each need is to YOU. Rate each one in Column A on a scale of 0–4 as follows:

0	1	2	3	4
not applicable	not important at all	a little important	somewhat important	very important

Second, consider how fully you believe each need is being met. In Column B, rate each one in terms of your satisfaction with the degree to which it is met on a scale of 0–4 as follows:

0	1	2	3	4
not applicable	very unsatisfied	usually unsatisfied	usually satisfied	very satisfied

	Column A	Column B

Economic

Making enough money
Having a good job
Managing the budget
Teaching children about money
Other:

_____

_____

Health and Security

Exercising
Eating right
Getting enough rest
Getting enough medical and
   dental care
Feeling free from danger
Other:

_____

_____

Physical

Cooking and eating meals
Taking care of clothes (laundry,
   mending, ironing, etc.)
Taking care of yourself (bathing,
   dressing, grooming, etc.)
Cleaning house
Having adequate transportation
Shopping
Making household repairs
Doing yard work
Other:

_____

_____

(continued)

	Column A	Column B

Recreation

Having interesting hobbies
Participating in sports
Having family fun
Just relaxing
Other:

_____

_____

Socialization

Being with family
Being with friends
Having close friends
Other:

_____

_____

Self-Definition

Knowing yourself
Feeling needed and worthwhile
Feeling content with who you are
Needing other people
Feeling good about job
Feeling good about home and
    family
Other:

_____

_____

Affection

Feeling loved
Expressing love
Having intimate relationships
Feeling satisfied with sexual
    intimacy
Other:

_____

_____

Education

Going to school (school,
    college, technical, etc.)
Learning new job skills
Learning new things in general
Other:

_____

_____

you have devised a few time-savers over the years. If you share these with friends, the chances are they will have a few ideas to exchange with you. Everybody is interested in saving time; it's the one commodity that is always in short supply.

You have already taken the first step recommended by many time management experts. Look back at your answers in Exercise 5A. Are there any needs you and others in your family agreed were unimportant? Now think back over the last week or so; did you spend time on these tasks? If you did, think about ways you could either cut out the activity or delegate it. There's no sense spending precious time on something nobody thinks is important.

The list of possible time-saving strategies is endless. You can tackle time management in a big way, with lists and calendars and special methods. If you're interested, you can find these methods described in the books suggested in the "Resources" appendix at the back of this book. But if a major overhaul of your use of time is not your style, you might still want to try one or more of the suggestions we have listed in Table 5.1.

THE POWER OF PEOPLE

Another way to meet some of your needs is to make better use of the resources you identified in Chapters 3 and 4. This is really a two-step process. First, consider what jobs members of your family and others in your social and professional network are doing now. Second, think about possible ways these tasks might be reallocated or other resources called into play.

Identifying who does which jobs in your family is not as easy as it may seem because it is not always possible to place a given activity in a single category. Families do not, of course, consciously tell themselves, "Now we are engaging in recreation; what fun!" or "Now it's time for a little education." Rather, a husband may hug his wife as they stand by the sink washing dishes. Or a father might give his teenage daughter a few pointers on boys as they work together repairing her stereo. Cuddling up to read a bedtime story fulfills recreational, educational, and affectional needs. Some needs, such as self-definition, are seldom directly addressed, but rather are met in the context of other activities. It is important to realize the family needs you are meeting in the course of day-to-day activities and interactions.

Because of the integrative way in which needs are met, your family may not be consciously aware of the many less tangible contributions that each member makes to others. You may be especially

Table 5.1. Time management tips

1. Recognize that inevitably some of your time will be spent on activities outside your control.
2. Don't waste time regretting your failures; concentrate on action steps to further your goals.
3. Don't waste time feeling guilty about what you don't do; concentrate on activities that yield the greatest long-term benefit.
4. Allow yourself to relax and "do nothing" for brief periods.
5. Try to enjoy whatever you are doing. Don't shortchange yourself during relaxation or work.
6. Before you start a task, ask yourself why you're doing it. If your answer is not convincing, do something else.
7. Schedule a regular 5–15 minute daily planning time to make a "to do" list of specific items.
8. Arrange "to do" items in order of priority.
9. Do first things first; train yourself to go down your "to do" list without skipping over difficult items.
10. Have confidence in your judgment of priorities, and stick to them in spite of difficulties.
11. Set *reasonable* timelines for yourself and others.
12. Try not to run only one errand at a time or go to the store for only one item; save up tasks to do once a week.
13. Take along some small tasks you can do if you need to be someplace where you'll have to wait (for example, the doctor's office).
14. If you can, delegate some responsibilities if they become too great. A little give-and-take with your support systems can go a long way.

unaware of the contributions of the disabled or ill member of your family. Often, we focus on the negative aspects of special needs. However, when asked about the *benefits* of having a disabled or chronically ill family member, most families are able to provide an answer. Most often those answers suggest that the member with a disability or illness best contributed to the affectional, self-definitional, and educational needs of other family members. As the mother of a woman with a physical disability said:

> She gave us great tolerance for being different. She gave us a lot of compassion and gave me a clearer picture of life.

The spouse of a physically disabled woman expressed similar feelings:

For the first time in my life I had to learn to talk about my feelings. It wasn't easy, by God, but it sure helped me realize that there was more to my wife, and to me, than what we do and how we do it. I'm learning to look at life from the inside-out.

Exercise 5B provides you with an opportunity to think about who is *currently* responsible for meeting needs in your family. As you fill it out, try to think of everyone's contribution. Even if some people only participate in a task once in a while, don't forget to list them.

As you completed Column A of this exercise, perhaps you found that your family members share fairly evenly in all tasks. Or you may have found that some people concentrate their energy in some areas but not in others. You may have also found that some people contribute more than others. There are an infinite variety of ways for families to divide their tasks among their members. No one way is the right way. As long as all family members are comfortable with the division of labor, everything's fine. If someone is dissatisifed, however, that's a different story. One person may think he or she has an unfair share of the family responsibilities. Or someone's needs in one or more areas may be unmet. Often, open communication can resolve the dissatisfaction. Perhaps the simple acts of filling out these exercises and talking about the results are enough to make changes. If not, then the issue can perhaps be resolved through problem solving. You might want to consider any unmet needs you found in Exercise 5A or any dissatisfaction with the way family responsibilities are allocated when we begin the problem-solving process in Chapter 7.

In Columns B and C of Exercise 5B, you may again have written a wide variety of answers. Perhaps you found the name of one friend turning up over and over as a source of help for many needs. Or you may rely on different friends for different sorts of help. The same pattern is true of professional support. Here, of course, your use of these resources depends on a combination of your family's preferences and values and the availability of different services in the community.

If you are interested in expanding your use of social and professional support, we encourage you to look at some of the suggestions in Chapters 3 and 4. In addition, Exercise 5C is designed to help you think of specific friends or agencies who might help with some of your unmet needs.

HOW NEEDS CHANGE

Just as values change over time, so do needs and the way they are met. We encourage you to keep the exercises in this chapter and look back

Exercise 5B

Below is a list of tasks commonly associated with meeting the needs listed in Exercise 5A. We have left some blanks for you to add any other tasks that are special to your family. You may also want to put "NA" beside any tasks your family does not do. In Column A, write the names or initials of ALL the members of your family who do these tasks. In Column B, write the names or initials of friends, neighbors, relatives, co-workers, or other people who help out with each task. Finally, in Column C, write the names or initials of any service agencies or professionals who provide help in that area. You might want to look back at Exercise 3A to jog your memory about the various people who make up your social and professional network.

	Column A (Family members)	Column B (Social support)	Column C (Professional support)

Economic
Making money
Managing the budget
Teaching children about money
Other:

_____

_____

Health and Security
Teaching children
   about diet and exercise
Providing medical,
   dental, and eye care
Providing security
Other:

_____

_____

Physical
Cooking and cleaning up
Cleaning house
Taking care of clothes
   (laundry, mending, etc.)
Grooming (bathing,
   dressing, etc.) small children,
   disabled or ill person
Driving and maintaining car
Shopping
Fixing things around the house
Doing yard work
Other:

_____

_____

Recreation
Helping other family
   members with hobbies
Playing games or sports
   with other family members
Going on or organizing outings
Relaxing around the
   house with family
Other:

_____

_____

(continued)

Exercise 5B
(continued)

	Column A	Column B	Column C

Socialization

Teaching family members
   to interact with others
Spending time with friends
Spending time with
   other family members
Talking/listening to others
Other:

_____

_____

Self-Definition

Expressing appreciation
   to other family members
Supporting other family
   members in their jobs
Supporting other
   family members in
   their role at home
Providing constructive
   feedback to other
   family members
Other:

_____

_____

Affection

Expressing affection

Expressing personal
   feelings to others
Initiating intimacy
Other:

_____

_____

Education

Helping other family
   members with homework
Supporting other family
   members in their education
Teaching skills to
   others (for example,
   cooking, car repair)
Teaching religious
   and/or other values
Teaching general
   knowledge to others
Other:

_____

_____

Exercise 5C

Below we have provided spaces for each of the eight broad areas of family needs. In the first column, think of people in your social support network (friends, relatives, neighbors, co-workers, etc.) who could be helpful in that area. Beside their names, jot down the specific way they can help. Do the same thing in the second column for professionals or agencies in your community. In both cases, try to think of people or agencies you did NOT include in that particular area of need in Exercise 5B. In other words, try to think of resources you are not using now. For example, one family had an aunt and uncle who lived nearby and a city recreation department. Their list of ways these supports could be helpful in the area of recreation is included as an example.

Recreation

Social supporters	Professional supporters
Aunt Helen—can take Joey to the park	*Rec. Dept.—we can enroll Joey in swimming class*

Economic needs

Social supporters	Professional supporters

Health and security needs

Social supporters	Professional supporters

Physical needs

Social supporters	Professional supporters

(continued)

Recreational needs

Social supporters _____   Professional supporters _____

Socialization needs

Social supporters _____   Professional supporters _____

Self-definition needs

Social supporters _____   Professional supporters _____

Affectional needs

Social supporters _____   Professional supporters _____

Educational needs

Social supporters _____   Professional supporters _____

over them a year from now. As we move through the life cycle—from childhood, to adolescence, and into the stages of adulthood—our needs change with the new demands of growth and development. Similarly, family priorities vary as members reach new developmental milestones. In families with young children, for instance, physical needs may occupy much of the family's time and energy. Families with adolescents may be more concerned with vocational choices and issues related to self-definition. Expression of affection with young children usually takes the form of physical contact, such as giving a tickle or a pat on the behind. But with adolescents, such expressions may be considered highly inappropriate, and expressions of affection must take other forms.

The changing nature of needs may pose problems for families with a disabled or chronically ill member. Depending again on the type and severity of the disability, a person may have some needs that are age-appropriate and some that are not. For example, a 15-year-old adolescent with a mental age of 8 may need a good deal more privacy than his or her parents initially perceive. The emerging sexuality of a disabled teenager is another often-cited issue that needs to be confronted. The physical care needs of a parent with a chronic illness may appear reminiscent of a young child's needs, requiring a parent-child reversal of roles.

The family must then cope with age-appropriate needs in some functions and age-discrepant needs in others. It is a difficult problem of perception, somewhat akin to rubbing one's stomach and patting one's head at the same time. In general, parents gradually encourage their children to meet their own needs as they become more capable of accepting responsibility (and as parents become increasingly worn out!). Families must determine for themselves the age at which they feel it is appropriate for children to assume such responsibility. What are the views in your own family on child versus adult roles? How does having a family member with a disability or illness affect these views?

One final point about needs that cannot be emphasized enough is that *all* family members have needs. In the past, professionals who worked with individuals having disabilities or illnesses advocated neglecting their needs in favor of the rest of the family by having them institutionalized. Now, professionals are more likely to demand that families organize their lives to give consistent first priority to addressing the needs of the disabled or ill person. Neither perspective is constructive or valid in our opinion. We believe that families should learn that everyone's needs are legitimate and that there are ways to balance those needs to reach an equitable arrangement. Families need practical, concrete suggestions on handling the daily needs and problems associated with living with, caring for, and loving a person with a disability or illness far more frequently than they need therapy. In Part II, we provide you with the means to address the unmet needs of your family. In particular, Chapter 7 is designed to help your family utilize the communication skills learned in Chapter 6 to express and identify your most pressing current needs and thus take the first and most fruitful step toward achieving these ends.

PART

II

PROBLEM SOLVING

In Part I, we looked at the many strengths your family can use to cope with the major and minor challenges of life. Your values, coping strategies, and the resources of people both inside and outside your family all form a deep wellspring of strength from which you can draw. In Part II, we show you how to take the strengths you already have and apply them to unmet needs or other problems you may face either now or in the future.

The format we are suggesting is a *problem-solving* model. A model, in the sense we are using it, provides an approach or system for accomplishing a goal. In this case, a problem-solving model is a step-by-step way of working through a problem. Problem solving is *active*, *systematic*, and *logical*, rather than impulsive, emotional, or passive. Many people do take a passive approach to problems; they decide to "wait and see" or hope the problem will go away. Sometimes this approach works, but often it limits options. For example, we interviewed an 82-year-old mother whose adult daughter with a mental disability was living with her at home. We asked about her plans for her daughter's future, and she told us:

> I don't have any. There aren't any [group] homes in this town that can serve Carol, because she has some medical problems. I don't want her in a nursing home, either. I have no idea what will happen when I'm gone. I suppose the Good Lord will provide.

No doubt this mother is correct—*someone* will make a decision about where Carol can live after her mother dies. Will that decision, made in a hurry and in the midst of sorrow over her mother's death, be the best one for Carol? Will Carol's needs be met in the best possible way? And is her mother really free from worry now? Maybe—but then again, maybe not. Carol's situation is one where some careful problem solving could be extremely helpful.

There are numerous problem-solving models used by a variety of people and organizations. Counselors use a version of problem solving to help their clients work through personal problems. Businesses use problem solving to help them overcome obstacles, design new products, or plan expansions. A problem-solving model can be a complex method filled with mathematical formulas and used by military planners to develop a global defense strategy. Or it can be a simple process used by a teacher to guide a class as it decides on a group science project. But even the most complex problem-solving model boils down into a few simple steps that all of us can use. These are the steps we are suggesting to you, as presented in Figure 2.

First, in order to solve a problem, we have to know what it is. This step is not always as easy as it seems. Some problems are actually several subproblems in one. They look overwhelming until we take them apart and look at each step. Also, there are ways to define a problem that make it easier to solve. Finally, most families are facing more than one problem at a time. The question is, which one should you solve first?

Once the problem is defined and a particular issue chosen, the next step is to think of all possible solutions. This is the step many families skip. They take the most obvious action or the one they have taken in the past. Brainstorming is the process of identifying as many solutions as possible. Brainstorming can and should be fun. It gives your family an opportunity to range far afield and come up with many creative possibilities that might seem—at first glance—almost crazy.

With a whole range of possibilities before you, the next step is to evaluate those alternatives and to choose the best one. This task involves using a number of yardsticks, or criteria, ranging from family values to practical considerations. It also involves trying to visualize the future consequences of each alternative.

The final step in problem solving is, of course, actually carrying out the solution you have chosen. This might mean simply doing what

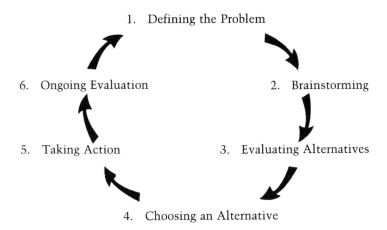

Figure 2. Steps in family problem solving.

everyone has decided. Or in the case of a more complicated solution, it might mean developing a step-by-step schedule, assigning specific tasks to different people, and setting deadlines for the accomplishment of each task. Taking action also involves checking to see how well the solution worked and, depending on the results, choosing a new alternative or tackling the next problem.

Just as in Part I, we have included several exercises in each chapter to help you think through the problem-solving process. We want to emphasize, however, that these exercises can be approached in many different ways. For example, you might write them out or talk them out in a special family discussion time. Or you might simply try out some of the activities after dinner or while taking a walk. Choose to do them in a way that fits your own individual family style. Certainly, the *last* thing we want to do is give you a new and time-consuming task that doesn't fit comfortably with your family's way of doing things. So, feel free to be flexible—do all or part of the exercises, discuss them with all or part of your family, write down your ideas, or just think about them. Experiment. The main purpose of this book is to help you sharpen your own personal problem-solving style. And that can't be done by following a rigid formula.

One final point is that an essential ingredient to successful *family* problem solving is good communication. Certainly, an individual could go through the problem-solving process with a minimum of communication with others. But we are talking about *family* problems in this book. We strongly believe that everyone's needs and opinions are important. And we also believe that what happens to one person in the family affects all the other family members to some degree. Therefore, successful problem solving requires that you communicate—talk *and* listen—as a family.

CHAPTER

6

Talking Things Out
Family Communication

Just as all families encounter problems, all families have the potential ability to work them through. However, we have found that one vital factor characterizes those families most successful at solving family problems: good communication. Good communication, once a buzzword of the 1960s, can mean many different things to many different people. To some, it might mean the ability to express oneself effectively or the process of setting aside time in which to discuss how things are going. To others, it might simply mean an appropriate and well-timed wink or a smile worth the proverbial thousand words. Good communication encompasses all these notions and more. The purpose of this chapter is not to tell you the right way to communicate, because human interaction involves such tremendous diversity that we would be foolish to attempt such a judgment. Rather, its purpose is to help you define your own family's style of communication and determine where you would like to improve or simply capitalize on your strengths. From there, we hope to help your family take advantage of these communication strengths so you can better use the problem-solving process. As you might already suspect, the process of cooperative family problem solving is intimately tied to the process of communication your family continually uses and develops.

Whether problem solving involves international politics, medical care for a child with cerebral palsy, or housing for an elderly couple with chronic illnesses, communication forms the foundation and the cement for reaching out and negotiating a resolution. Communication, first and foremost a natural and essential human skill, is a process in which we all engage to greater or lesser degrees of satisfaction. Because of the extent of human differences, communication styles are infinitely diverse. However, as our own experience has taught us, certain styles of communication feel more appropriate, pleasing, and helpful than others. That is, we have a sense of what forms of communication are most effective for accomplishing our goals. We have all had the experience of discussing a concern or problem with someone. In these instances, we may remember the interaction as particularly rewarding and helpful or particularly disappointing and unpleasant. These responses correspond to our individual perceptions of good communication. Exercise 6A will help you identify communication elements that have been either particularly helpful and pleasant or unhelpful and aversive to you in the past.

We all have our own expectations of how others can best respond to our needs and how we can best respond to the needs of others. Caring, directness, honesty, reason, sensitivity, and a sense of humor are all vehicles for effective communication. Yet, whatever our style, how we choose to express ourselves and interact with others is vitally important to the successful resolution of our needs, be they affectional, physical, or financial. The following discussion is designed to enable you to identify and attain your own preferred style of communicating with others.

HOLISTIC SELF-EXPRESSION: USING HEART AND MIND

In addition to the daily thoughts, experiences, and affections we communicate to family members, a variety of needs, concerns, problems, and conflicts can also spark family communication. How family members choose to express these thoughts and feelings can have a profound impact on whether the intended message is accurately received and whether a resolution is attained. For example, failing to express a need for more affection greatly decreases the likelihood that it will be met. That failure often results in an "If I'd only known" refrain. Or conveying one's need for affection through hostile words and accusations similarly obscures the true message and makes resolution more difficult. Thus, particularly when problems need to be

Exercise 6A

1. Recall a situation in which you felt particularly let down and disappointed after having discussed a concern or problem with someone.

    What did the person say that disappointed you?

    _____

    What didn't he or she say?

    _____

    What was most unhelpful about the interaction?

    _____

    How might you have contributed to this unhelpful experience?

    _____

    What would you do differently in the future?

    _____

    How did you feel about the problem afterwards?

    _____

2. Now think of a situation in which you felt particularly pleased and assisted by another person with whom you discussed a problem or concern.

    What did the person do or say that made communication clear and easy?

    _____

    What was most helpful about his or her manner or response?

    _____

    What did you do to contribute to the success of this interaction?

    _____

    How did you feel about the problem afterwards?

    _____

resolved, good communication can be a family's greatest asset. Such communication involves an awareness of both feelings and sensibilities (that is, thoughts), making room for your own special style of conveying both heart and mind in one message.

Where needs and problems are concerned, emotions often run high in family communications. Anger, fear, sorrow, hope, and anticipation can all make direct, rational communication difficult. The tendency is often to shoot from the hip or, in this case, from the heart. For many, this spontaneous and emotional style has been successful. For others, it has been met with resistance, conflict, or unsuccessful problem resolution. For these individuals, the greatest asset of their emotional strength and investment can be maximized by additional contributions of thought. If emotions can be likened to the speed and stamina of a racecar driver, rational forethought can be likened to the same driver's winning concentration and technique. Without each element, the driver is lost, and his or her best intentions are either stuck motionless in the pit or dashed uncontrollably against a barrier. Thus, in communicating a message, it is often helpful to maintain a holistic approach, combining resources of both the heart and mind. Tempering your feelings with some analysis and thought or, conversely, freeing your mental rehearsal with an open expression of emotions can help to keep communication on a steady, secure, and smooth track. The collaboration of heart and mind helps maximize your emotional and mental resources. It enables you to convey a need, problem, or feeling in a clear, direct, and easy-to-receive fashion.

One way to determine whether or not a message successfully combines heart and mind is to determine whether it is *constructive* or *destructive* in nature. As the terms imply, constructive messages build communication, whereas destructive messages break it down. When your goal is to resolve a problem, constructive communication is particularly effective in building both an emotional and a working alliance. How can a family effectively combine heart and mind messages into constructive communication?

Fortunately, your family already has all the necessary tools for communicating constructively. Simply put, this type of good communication involves expressing needs and feelings in a clear, direct, and nonthreatening manner. Such communication is generally calm and rational, yet still intimately tied to the emotions from which it arises. That is, we are not advocating a robot-like message devoid of human feeling and need. Rather, we suggest that constructive communication involves each individual's ability to capture feelings with a unique combination of heart and mind messages. Such a combination is generally nonthreatening, honest, and responsible, but varies in its degree and balance of emotionality and rationality. The following example helps illustrate this point.

Edith and Joe Salkowitz have been married for 10 years. Two years ago, Edith developed breast cancer and immediately underwent a radical mastectomy. The surgeon deemed the operation a success, stating that Edith had a good, although not 100%, chance of avoiding a future bout with cancer.

Traumatized by the threat to her life that the cancer posed, as well as the damage to her feminine body image, Edith has been understandably distraught. Joe, sensitive to his wife's fears and insecurity, has sought to support her as much as possible. However, having had his own fears of loss and death ignited by Edith's cancer, Joe has been unable to maintain the same closeness they enjoyed in the past. In fact, Edith finds his hugs rather empty, sexual contact at a minimum, and conversations carefully steered away from sensitive topics.

Unaware of Joe's fears of death and of losing her, Edith has assumed that his distance stems from disenchantment or even repulsion over her mastectomy. She feels sexually undesirable and unfeminine as it is, and Joe's lack of intimate emotional or sexual interest only confirms her worst fears. She feels a mixed assortment of agonizing emotions: anger, hurt, panic, and grief. She feels close to the end of her emotional reserves. Edith realizes that she must talk with Joe in the hope of resolving their problems or at least reaching a better understanding and connection between them. Her only question is how to express her feelings: "What should I say?"

Edith clearly has many options regarding how best to communicate with her husband. She is emotionally stressed, yet she feels that her needs are so important that she does not want to threaten or confuse Joe and thus risk reducing their chances of building an alliance and eventual resolution. Although her gut emotional reaction is to yell at Joe—"You don't love me anymore! You find me disgusting without breasts!"—she thinks for a moment about more constructive, less threatening messages that combine less heart and more mind. Her next thought is to temper her emotions slightly with reason: "I know that I am no longer the woman you married. I am unattractive, and while I can't blame you, I feel terrible that you will never be able to love me as before." But Edith realizes that she is "mind reading—talking for Joe before he has even had the opportunity to express himelf. Thus, Edith decides to first determine what her feelings are and then to simply express them to Joe in as clear and uncomplicated a form as possible. This, she decides, will give him the freedom to respond spontaneously and nondefensively, providing her with valuable, honest feedback.

Edith determines that, first, she feels unattractive and unlovable to the man she loves. This makes her fear of death all the more lonely and frightening. The simple truth of these feelings strikes her *as the best message she could possibly convey. So, after asking Joe to set aside some time for an important talk, she says, "Joe, I have been struggling with a lot of feelings that I need to share with you. Mainly, I have been feeling terribly unattractive and unlovable since my surgery. I have an awful fear of losing your affection and support when I need it most. All this has made the thought of cancer all the more devastating." Given this clear, honest, nonthreatening entrée, Joe was able to similarly express his own thoughts and feelings. By constructively speaking with their own combinations of heart and mind, Edith and Joe were able to better understand each other's needs and begin, together, the process of meeting them.*

Several key points are illustrated by Edith's struggle to communicate important needs effectively. First, it is important when combining heart and mind messages to be sure it is your own heart and mind that is being expressed! Edith was able to catch herself when she sensed that she was about to tell Joe what *his* feelings were. Wisely, she refocused her attention on areas that she knew best: her own thoughts and feelings.

Second, many of the emotions that accompanied her damaged self-image, such as anger and blame, were recognized by Edith as being potentially destructive. That is, they threatened to break down communication if expressed as the primary message in their raw form. Thus, Edith was able to focus on her deeper needs in order to best convey her message, calling on mental resources to help capture her emotions. This action subsequently allowed Joe the opportunity to respond in kind—openly, honestly, and with both heart and mind. At a later point, once communication is established, it will be easier for Edith to express her important angry feelings to Joe: "Boy, sometimes I felt so angry at you when I thought you were abandoning me!"

Third, Edith learned that the simple, honest, direct expression of her feelings was best conveyed in a calm, responsible, and nonthreatening fashion. By taking responsibility for her feelings and not casting blame, Edith succeeded in building communication. And, by tempering her strong emotions with knowledge of both Joe's sensitivities and the importance of the issue, Edith was able to successfully convey a constructive message. Thus, the Salkowitz's case illustrates the beauty of good communication: It is straightforward and merges aspects of each individual's heart and mind, capitalizing on the unique emotional and mental strengths of the communicators.

For some practice using heart and mind messages, try doing Exercise 6B. Have each member of your family complete this exercise, and compare your responses.

Exercise 6B

Consider the following example:

> Joyce Wethers is a single mother whose 3-year-old son James has been
> diagnosed as autistic. For weeks, Joyce has been trying to locate a satisfac-
> tory educational program for James, but to no avail. Despite numerous
> telephone calls, Joyce feels that she has gotten the "runaround," and she
> wonders if there is any justice at all for children with disabilities. Frustrated
> and angry, Joyce decides to contact the superintendent of the public school
> system directly, both to express her need and to attain some assistance.
> Before picking up the receiver, she pauses and considers what to say.

How might Joyce best communicate her needs and concerns to the
superintendent? Put yourself in Joyce's place, and write what you would
say:

_____

_____

_____

Below, check the styles of communication you incorporated into your
message:

_____ Used more heart than mind
_____ Used more mind than heart
_____ Used equal balance of heart and mind
_____ Assumed responsibility
_____ Imposed blame
_____ Included threats
_____ Straightforwardness
_____ Presented calmly
_____ Avoided mind reading
_____ Will likely build communication (would be constructive if
          spoken to me)

What were the best aspects of your message?

_____

_____

What aspects of your message would you change?

_____

_____

BENDING AN EAR . . . OR TWO

When we have invested heart and mind in conveying an important message, being understood can be wonderfully satisfying. Yet, although we may sometimes feel that our message has been well received and acknowledged, at other times our message seems to fall on deaf ears, and communication screeches to a halt. What enables us to feel that our message has been heard and our communication successful?

Active listening is the key to the two-way flow that makes up communication. Active listening is a special way of attending to and acknowledging that you have heard another person's message. Central to active listening are three components: 1) paying attention to the person with whom you are interacting, 2) checking out and confirming your understanding of what the other person is saying, and 3) accepting the person's right to his or her own feelings and beliefs. Although these components are self-explanatory, they may also seem deceptively simple. Let's look at each of these components more closely.

Paying Attention

All of us who have feared giving a speech to a sleeping audience or expressing an important concern to an uninterested loved one understand the fundamental importance of paying attention. There are many ways to pay attention, and naturally we all have our own styles. Some listen with expressive eyes and sympathetic "uh huhs." Others divert their eyes and acknowledge their understanding with knowing nods of the head. What is important here is not only that the listener attends carefully to the speaker but also that the listener is able to *demonstrate* that he or she is indeed paying close attention. That is, although we may actually be able to hear someone with the television turned up and the newspaper in hand, we are unlikely to be convincing in our role as active listener! Thus, letting people know that they have our attention is far different from simply listening. Active listening demands responsiveness—signals or messages of our own that tell the speaker that he or she is being heard. Such signals can involve eye contact, nods of the head, verbal acknowledgments, knowing touches, or various other individual and highly personal gestures. Some styles are so ingrained and natural that they escape our conscious planning entirely. Exercise 6C will help you get in touch with your own listening style.

Exercise 6C

1. How do you feel others know that you are paying attention? How successful do you feel you are in letting others know that they are being heard?

2. Ask another family member the following questions:
   a. How well do you feel I pay attention to you when you speak?
   b. How do you know that I am paying attention (what signs do I give you)?

3. What did you learn about your listening skills? List below those aspects that you would like to change or emphasize even more:

_____   _____
_____   _____
_____   _____

Yes, I Understand

As you listen attentively to another person, the next important aspect of listening is to confirm that you understand the message. As you well know, not all messages combine heart and mind in a way that makes responding easy. Particularly where strong emotions are involved, it is often difficult to hear exactly what is being communicated. For example, in trying to express a need for greater independence, an adolescent with arthritis might say, "You won't give me any room; you treat me like a little kid! I am leaving tomorrow; I have got to get out on my own." One way to check out your understanding is to simply ask for clarification: "I'm not sure I understand what it is you want right now. Are you saying that you need more freedom at home or out on your own?" Asking questions directed at uncovering the central message (the calm eye of the tornado) not only improves your understanding but also is a way of saying that you care, you are listening, and are trying very hard to understand. This type of message can often go a long way toward calming emotions and making heart-and-mind communication possible.

Another way to confirm your understanding is to restate or paraphrase what you have just understood to be the person's message. For example, if Shawn says, "All this physical therapy is driving me absolutely crazy," a paraphrased response might sound something like this: "It sounds like you are really frustrated with your therapy." At this point, Shawn can either say, "Yes, all that work is not paying off," or clarify her message further: "Well, not really frustrated, but tired of being so absorbed in my disability." This type of active listening creates a back-and-forth flow of communication. The listener in this example has succeeded in gaining a clearer picture of Shawn's feelings and has opened the door for a continuing process of successful communication. Exercise 6D will help you practice the communication strategy of paraphrasing.

Accepting the Individuality of Family Members

Perhaps the most difficult aspect of successful active listening is accepting the right of others to feel and believe as they wish. Often, when we disagree with another person's viewpoint, we have an urge to argue, criticize, or convert. Although there is a place for this type of debate, in family problem solving it is important to keep in mind that active listening can help other members feel accepted. Active listening creates an atmosphere in which new ideas and diverse opinions

---

Exercise 6D

Assume that the following messages are directed at you. As an active listener, paraphrase each message in order to check out your understanding.

Example: "Don will never be able to take care of himself—his future is hopeless."

Response: "It sounds like you are feeling hopeless about Don's future."

Message 1: "I just can't do it all on my own anymore. I just can't stand it!"

Response 1:

Message 2: "Our sex life is nonexistent. You must not really love me anymore."

Response 2:

Message 3: "Nobody cares what I want. I might as well not even be part of a family."

Response 3:

---

can be freely expressed. It can thus ensure that all available options are considered and a good solution determined. But first, members must feel that they have the right to express themselves. This is where you, as an active listener, come in. Because few of us persist in a struggle to communicate our thoughts and feelings to a listener who does not accept our right to our own views, active listening is often needed to establish an atmosphere where communication is rewarding and expressive.

It is important to point out here that accepting others' rights to their own beliefs does not mean that we also agree with their point of view. Rather, such acceptance simply reflects our respect for their individuality—for their right to be themselves. This form of acceptance can go a long way toward building communication. The speaker is not put on the defensive by attempts to change him or her, and the listener is in turn better able to freely express his or her own views. Thus, communication is established in the form of a round table give-and-take family discussion that is particularly well suited to family problem solving.

These same principles apply when communication must be carried out long distance, particularly by phone. Often we need to discuss issues with people we cannot meet with in person. Family members are often scattered across the country; resource persons often live in distant towns. In such cases, we may avoid contacts or may accumulate huge and unnecessary bills if our phone communication is ineffective. If long distance communication is an issue for you, use the tips suggested in Table 6.1.

SUMMARY

In our discussions of heart-and-mind communication and active listening, we have tried to convey a number of important points about family communication. First and foremost is the message that we can all determine the individual manner in which we choose to communicate. Some of us communicate in a more emotional fashion; others rely on their rational powers. As observed by one woman with diabetes:

> My husband doesn't communicate much, and my dad likes people who can say as much with as few words as possible. But me, I'm expressive and love to talk!

Whatever our style, it is the combination of heart and mind that makes our messages uniquely effective. An awareness of the con-

Table 6.1. Tips for long distance communication

1. Decide what you want to accomplish *first*. You may even want to list the issues you expect to cover or the information you hope to obtain before picking up the phone.
2. Know what you want from the other person and articulate that need, whether you want input into a decision or simply emotional support and understanding.
3. Be selective about what you expect to gain from the other. Capitalize on people's strengths, and avoid demanding what others cannot give.
4. Develop a common understanding of the problem.
5. Establish a phone budget, and divide your allotted time into segments. Assign specific, manageable tasks to each phone call.
6. Realize that you may have differences in your approach to a problem and in your feelings about it. But be sure to articulate those differences.
7. Be tenacious. Don't hang up! It is too easy to shut others out long distance and avoid communication. Stay in touch, and express your willingness to get past angry feelings and differences of opinion.
8. Don't assume anything. Words can take on different meanings by phone; ask for clarification and explanation.
9. Writing letters may be more economical. Some people are better able to communicate in writing.
10. Emphasizing mind over heart messages can often facilitate the expeditious exchange of information.
11. Be prepared to *listen*, as well as speak. Establish confidence and trust in each other.
12. Shop around for competitive long distance phone rates!

tributions of heart and mind in our own messages can be invaluable to our ability to communicate in the manner we prefer.

In delivering messages, we can often ask ourselves, "If this message was spoken to me, would it build or break down communication?" Your intuition is probably the best indicator of whether your message will be constructive or destructive.

In bending an ear to the words of others, we can respond in our own unique styles of paying attention, confirming our understanding of the message, and acknowledging others' rights to feel as they do. With practice as good communicators—that is, effective message senders and receivers—you should be beautifully prepared to tackle family problems. The following chapter discusses both the first step in family problem solving—defining the problem—and how your communication skills can be further developed to define and express even the most sensitive and urgent of family problems.

CHAPTER

7

Defining the Problem

The needs of family members can seem endless. Fortunately, most of these needs are met regularly in the course of daily activities. As crucial as they might be, these adequately met needs are not the focus of our attention. As mentioned in Chapter 5, the needs that contribute to family and personal difficulties are those that go *unmet.* Unmet needs are those that grow, fester, and rarely disappear without active attention. It is these *unmet needs* that are best defined as *problems* targeted for active resolution.

Should all needs be immediately identified and expressed? No! All families cannot deal effectively with all their needs at one time. Although families may need to be aware of these needs so they can be prepared to face them later, it is unrealistic to expect families to confront future or less urgent needs as consistently and actively as more current, pressing ones. As the parents of a 14-year-old boy with multiple disabilities said, "We take one day at a time. We can't handle *thinking about* age 21." This chapter is designed to help families deal with current unmet needs and to identify those unmet needs that demand immediate attention.

Many of us are reluctant to express our needs to other family members. Parents with ill or disabled children or spouses of ill or disabled adults may be particularly unwilling to do so. Drawing attention to our wants, desires, and conflicts feels selfish, aggressive, or burdensome. We feel that others are more important or that we have no right to ask for more than we already have or can obtain on our own. In the past, we have resented individuals who *demanded* that others meet their needs, and we may fear being perceived in the same way. These attitudes are both powerful and deeply engrained, yet they are neither realistic nor healthy. Why?

As discussed earlier, the needs of family members overlap considerably. That is, one member's need inevitably affects other members in one way or another. Consider the following example:

Sara Tahashi is the mother of four. Her oldest daughter, Jennifer, is 14 years old. Jennifer has been ill with anorexia nervosa for the past year, and Sara has felt heavily involved with Jennifer's meals, doctors, psychologists, and daily bouts of depression. Sara's husband, Sam, works full time and is not available during the day to help Sara manage Jennifer's crises, offer support, or to help with the household responsibilities.

Sara has felt the strain of her responsibilities at home becoming almost unbearable in the past year. The fear that her daughter may starve herself amidst plenty, as well as the constant stress of observing Jennifer's pain, confusion, and rituals, has taken a toll on Sara's energy and ability to cope. Furthermore, she feels that she has no time for herself and sees no respite ahead. Recently, Sara has become uncharacteristically irritable. Inside, she feels overworked and unfairly burdened with housework, child care, and Jennifer's needs; yet she feels guilty about expressing her intense need for relief. Sara has always considered herself competent and independent, and she attributes her pressing need for help to a weak and selfish failure on her part. Instead of expressing her needs, Sara finds herself snapping at Sam for no apparent reason, nagging the children, and having explosive fights with Jennifer. Although it is obvious to Sam that Sara is overwrought and unhappy, he does not completely understand why. The younger children, on the other hand, do not understand Sara's irritability and attribute her anger to something they have done. Jennifer considers herself the source of all her own, as well as her family's, grief and wonders if suicide is the only way out of her dilemma.

Sam has tried to talk with Sara about what is troubling her, but she merely says, "it's Jennifer," and tearfully rejects his attempts to listen and help. The children try to avoid her as much as possible, which only contributes to her sense of isolation and overwhelming responsibility. Thus, although Sara is struggling with personal unmet needs, the entire Tahashi family is strongly affected by what might be called the "fallout" from an unmet need.

As the case of the Tahashi family illustrates, ignoring an unmet need can be highly destructive to the well-being of the entire family. As one mother of a son with a physical disability said:

> You have to express your feelings. If you don't, you can become a martyr. And then nobody can win. It's a trap that families get into.

The message, then, is that it is both our *right*, as well as our *responsibility*, to express our needs. Not only does this expression accomplish the most important step in the process of solving problems but it also provides direct and honest information about family tensions to others. In the case of the Tahashi family, chances are that if Sara had expressed her need for more help, at least four positive outcomes would have been possible: 1) she may have avoided creating other problems; 2) she may have increased the probability of getting the help she desperately needed; 3) other family members may have been able to understand her angry behavior as stemming from her unmet needs, rather than feeling responsible themselves; and 4) Sara may have been forced to confront her involvement and identification with Jennifer's personal struggle. Therefore, expressing a need can have many positive effects, the most important of which are eventually resolving problems and minimizing negative fallout. Recall an unmet need you have had that you were hesitant to express. What feelings and thoughts kept you from expressing that need? Did other problems arise as a result of withholding it? Did you eventually express it? Why? What was the outcome? Would other family members be willing to answer these same questions?

EXPRESSING NEEDS CONSTRUCTIVELY

Of course, there are many ways to express a need. We have all had experiences when someone has angrily demanded that we meet their needs. Quite possibly we either refused, did so begrudgingly, or whispered a few curses under our breath. On the other hand, we have undoubtedly had a loved one express their needs to us in a manner to which we felt willing and able to respond. In what important ways do these styles of expressing needs differ? Consider the Tahashis' case for a moment. Sara could have expressed her need in any one of a number of *destructive* or *constructive* ways. The following are four examples of destructive statements:

1. "All of you are selfish and irresponsible!"
2. "I'm just upset about everything and everyone."
3. "None of you care about my needs."
4. "You all expect me to do everything around here!"

Now consider the following four constructive need statements. Perhaps you can note important differences.

1. "I am terribly unhappy because I feel that I need more help with the housework and with coping with my feelings about Jennifer."
2. "I feel so much pressure and responsibility that I know I need a break."
3. "I need some help with the house and with being there for Jennifer."
4. "I need more time for myself, but my responsibilities are just too demanding."

Why did we label the first four statements as being "destructive"? Need statements can be destructive in several ways. First, statements that cast blame on others are destructive because they tend to put others off and fail to express the need clearly, merely expressing a lot of residual anger instead. Second, statements that are vague about the precise nature of the need are difficult to address. If someone is "upset about everything," for instance, the listener has few clues about the source of the person's needs. Third, expressions that include "you" statements, but no "I" statements, usually fail to assume responsibility for one's feelings and needs. Thus, it is important when expressing needs to: 1) not attribute blame to others and thus avoid making other people the problem, 2) specify the nature of the need, and 3) include an "I" statement as a means of owning the need and its accompanying feelings.

These three positive elements of a constructive need statement deserve elaboration. First, as you can see in the examples of constructive statements, each includes an "I" statement. Saying "I really need and miss the affection we once shared" or "I am so stressed by work that something has to change" clarifies that the individual accepts responsibility for his or her feelings and needs. Second, positive need statements identify the nature of the need. Global statements, such as "I am fed up with the whole world" or "nothing ever works out for me," fail to identify a specific need. Such statements are positive in that they convey feeling, but they fall short of productively defining a need. Third, constructive need statements do not attribute blame to others. Although we might often feel that others play an important role in either meeting or creating given needs, we have the ultimate responsibility for defining and addressing our needs. By not making other people the causes of our problems, we avoid the trap of trying to change others to suit our needs. Perhaps most important, by avoiding the use of blame, we are more apt to enlist the support and understanding of others in meeting our needs. Consider the following case study:

Janice and Al Stern have been married for 18 years. They have two sons; David, age 9, and Charlie, age 15. Two years ago, Janice was severely burned in a gasoline fire at work. She suffered second- and third-degree burns over 50% of her body. As a result, she lost the functional use of her right arm and right eye, as well as most facial sensation. In addition to the loss of function, Janice has been deeply traumatized by the extensive cosmetic damage that makes her look, in her words, like "a freakish monster."

Over the past 4 months since returning from the hospital, Janice has surprised her family by becoming increasingly irritable, depressed, and hostile, despite improvement in her condition and lessening of the pain. She criticizes her children and husband for minor flaws, rebuffs their attempts at conversation, and generally experiences and exudes misery.

Recently, other family members have exhibited difficulties as well. Charlie has become involved in drug and alcohol abuse, frequently returning home late at night in a drunk and angry state. According to reports from his grade school, David has become uncharacteristically withdrawn, lethargic, and inattentive. At home, as well, the Sterns have been struggling with an atmosphere of tension and unhappiness that finally led them to heed the advice of a close relative and seek family counseling.

After several weeks of family therapy sessions, the Sterns became more able to express their troubling unmet needs. It gradually came out that much of Janice's anger and depression stemmed from her belief that her family found her physically repulsive and would never be able to grant her the same affections she valued so deeply in the past. With this information in the open, the Sterns were able to discuss Janice's physical appearance and convey their continued affection for her. In addition, Al, Charlie, and David were able to convey in their own way a continued need for her affection. After several tearful sessions where false beliefs and honest feelings were exposed, Janice became more able to express her needs directly and then to accept the subsequent affections her sons and husband sincerely felt. As a result, Janice felt less hopeless about the implications of her disability, and she resumed the physical and verbal contact with her family that comprised a need central to her sense of self-worth and overall well-being. Subsequently, David began to resume his normal activities with vigor, and Charlie's behavior became less destructive.

This example highlights several important points. First, allowing a need to go unmet does not make it disappear. More often than not, it merely festers and finds expression in undesirable outlets, such as despair or unprovoked hostility. Second, when one family member's needs are unfulfilled, there can be an equally disruptive effect on other family members. In the case of the Sterns, Janice's unmet affectional needs not only contributed to the general unhappiness of other members but also decreased their ability to meet their own affectional needs as well. Thus, a domino chain of confusion and conflict can often be set into motion when an unmet need is denied expression and, consequently, fulfillment. An unmet need, then, can rapidly turn into a "problem." Third, once a need is expressed responsibly, clearly, and without blame, it can have many positive effects on the entire family. It can open the lines of communication so that others can feel free to express their own feelings and needs. It can also mobilize the family to take action toward meeting the need or resolving the problem. Exercise 7A is designed to help you formulate and try out constructive and destructive need statements.

RESPONDING TO THE NEEDS OF OTHERS

Just as there are constructive and destructive ways to express needs, so are there positive and negative ways to receive and respond to the need statements of others. As the previous examples illustrated, it is easier to respond to a statement that is not blameful, vague, or irresponsible. It is helpful, however, to be equipped to transform even the most negative statement into a highly constructive one.

Exercise 7A

Think of a need you have been aware of during the past month. List three destructive need statements and then three constructive need statements to convey that need. Choose the best statement and try it out on a family member. How did he or she react?

NEED: _____

Three destructive need statements:

1. _____
2. _____
3. _____

Three constructive need statements:

1. _____
2. _____
3. _____

Best statement:

_____

Individuals express their needs to others for a variety of reasons. Perhaps they merely want a sympathetic ear or a sounding board off which to "bounce" their feelings. In other cases, an individual might be directly asking for help in resolving the need. As a listener, it is important to be aware of your role as recipient of the need statement and then to respond in an appropriate and constructive manner. The catch, however, is that "approriate" varies with each situation. Thus, it is a skillful individual who can cope effectively with the varied need statements he or she encounters daily.

The following suggestions can be helpful to you as you seek to deal effectively with the needs of family members. First, avoid becoming defensive. Although it is difficult to avoid launching a counterattack to a blameful need statement, it is helpful to remember that such blame stems from the strain of an unmet need. In other words, it might be helpful not to take such blame personally. Thus, taking one step backward into an objective position can be the first step toward avoiding unproductive conflict and proceeding to the heart of the matter: defining the unmet need. Second, try to gain a clear sense of the need or problem by asking the individual to clarify his or her statement. Often, paraphrasing the person's statement to check out your understanding is a useful technique. By restating the major points of a statement, it is possible to clarify and confirm that you understand the key messages. A natural tendency might be to respond to a need statement with a suggestion or with advice. It is important, however, to first make sure you have accurately heard what the person is saying. Third, try to refocus on the individual's needs even though you, or others, may be included in the need statement. Consider the following examples of positive responses to even the most destructive need statements.

Statement: You are selfish and never think of my needs!
Response: I'd like to understand your needs better. Tell me what need you are finding unfulfilled.

Statement: You are all slobs and expect me to do all the work of picking up after you!
Response: What I hear you saying is that you are angry because you feel you need more help with the housework.

Statement: I'm not a kid anymore! You think you can barge in here anytime!
Response: Would it help for us to think of ways to satisfy your need for more privacy?

Statement: I hate this wheelchair! It's ruining my entire life!
Response: What do you need that your wheelchair keeps you from getting?

Clearly, a great deal of patience is used in all these situations. Nobody likes to be attacked or hit with a barrage of angrily presented needs. The simple fact is that we are all human and have our own feelings. What can be a helpful strategy, however, is disarming the needy person's attack by *positively restating* his or her need. This serves the highly constructive purpose of conveying that the individual's needs are acknowledged, understood, and considered important. Few people persist in anger once they perceive that somebody understands them and that help is on the way. Exercise 7B can give your family practice in both expressing unmet needs and in paraphrasing those need statements in a constructive manner.

DEFINING A PROBLEM

By now, you should be ready to take your need statements and listening skills one step further. Once a need is expressed, it must be defined in a solvable form for active problem solving to proceed. That is, in order to resolve needs, it is often important that they be redefined in a more specific and objective form. At this point, we call such statements *problem definitions.*

Generally, the term "problem" connotes a negative situation, one to best be avoided in fact. Problems may call to mind images of stress, aggravation, obstacles, and stumbling blocks. It is not our intention here to view problems only in that negative way. Rather, we believe that by specifying a need in terms of a problem statement, a very positive step has been taken: The need has been identified and targeted for resolution. A problem is thus something we work out, much like an arithmetic problem. Although we may prefer to do other things than our math homework, solving problems enables us to get on with those things we value. Thus, we want to convey the belief that problems are merely needs or situations targeted for active resolution.

Exercise 7B

Gather your family together, picking a time that is most comfortable for everyone. Have each member take a turn expressing two unmet needs he or she is currently experiencing within the family. Express each need with an "I" statement, specifying the nature of the need and without attributing blame or responsibility to others. Similarly, try to listen to each other without defensiveness or argument. (If you can't think of any unmet needs, refer to the checklist you completed in Chapter 5.)

Finally, paraphrase each member's need statements in a constructive manner in order to check out the accuracy of the family's understanding. Have one member record each need statement and the accompanying paraphrased response in the spaces provided. Here are three examples of need statements and paraphrased responses:

Need Statement: I need to feel less overwhelmed by all the demands on my time and energy.

Paraphrase: You seem to feel like it's hard for you to set priorities for everything you feel like you need to do.

Need Statement: I hate to take my pills everyday.

Paraphrase: It sounds like you are really feeling how hard it is to live with an illness.

Need Statement: I need more money from somewhere to pay for the medicine and equipment I need.

Paraphrase: Maybe we could all put our heads together and try to figure out better ways to get your health-related needs paid for.

(continued)

Exercise 7B

(continued)

1. Need statement: _____

   _____

   Paraphrase: _____

   _____

2. Need statement: _____

   _____

   Paraphrase: _____

   _____

3. Need statement: _____

   _____

   Paraphrase: _____

   _____

4. Need statement: _____

   _____

   Paraphrase: _____

   _____

5. Need statement: _____

   _____

   Paraphrase: _____

   _____

6. Need statement: _____

   _____

   Paraphrase: _____

   _____

SEPARATING FEELINGS FROM ACTIONS

Although feelings are an integral and important aspect of every problem we encounter, in order to best take action, problem definitions should focus on action, rather than feelings. For example, consider the following need statement: "I have been depressed because I have been unable to sustain a relationship with a woman." By focusing on the concrete and action-oriented goal of sustaining an intimate relationship, the problem is defined in a way that makes it possible for you to develop strategies for attaining this goal. By focusing on actions, the problem is refined to its most solvable form. The following example illustrates this aspect of defining a problem.

Carlos Silva was a physical education instructor at a small rural high school for 18 years. One year ago, Carlos suffered a heart attack, and since then, he has fought a long and difficult battle against heart disease. Carlos's life-style has drastically changed in the wake of his advanced atherosclerosis because of his need to control his diet, exercise, and stress level. The loss of Carlos's rewarding and challenging job as a high school basketball coach has added insult to injury.

Carlos is troubled by feelings of frustration, depression, and worthlessness. Most days, he watches television. An avid sports fan, he also reads extensive sports literature and news. Carlos perceives that he is deeply frustrated by being unable to fulfill his great love of participating in sports. He misses coaching, as well as playing basketball, and has experienced a tremendous loss of self-esteem and enjoyment of life. Carlos expressed his needs to a former colleague. He stated that he felt miserable sitting at home all the time and missed coaching a great deal. After sorting through his feelings and thoughts, Carlos was able to clearly define his most pressing need in a solvable problem statement: "I need to become involved in sports again in one capacity or another."

With the problem so defined, Carlos had created a manageable situation. Given the clear goal of becoming involved in sports, Carlos would be able to begin gathering information and, eventually, generating alternatives for achieving this end. Defining a problem in terms of actions can thus be a constructive first step toward resolving an unmet need.

Another point that makes problem definition easier is this: Never include a solution in the definition. That is, in defining a need, it is best not to go beyond that point by prematurely suggesting a resolution. The goal of problem definition is to specify precisely what needs to be solved. For example, instead of Carlos saying, "I need to get my old job back," it is more productive, in the long run, for him to simply define the problem: "I need to become active in some aspect of sports again." This leaves the door open for him to pursue a variety of alternatives, including many of which he may be presently unaware. Similarly, instead of an individual saying, "I need the independent living center to transport me to my job every morning," it is more productive to define the problem as "I need transportation to work." Thus, problem definition should never include problem resolution. Instead, a clear statement of the need in solvable action-oriented form is the overriding goal of this phase of the problem-solving process. Exercise 7C is designed to help you restate your unmet needs as problem definitions.

Exercise 7C

Look over the list of need statements generated by family members in Exercise 7B. Select two for each family member, and restate each one as a solvable problem definition. That is, state each one in such a way that solutions are not included in the definition and specific actions comprise the focus of the statement. Save a copy of these problem definitions for later use. Here are some sample need statements and accompanying solvable problem definitions:

Need Statement	Solvable Problem Definition
Example A: I need more money for medicine and equipment.	I need a plan to figure out how I can get the medicine and equipment I need.
Example B: I need to feel less overwhelmed by work.	I need to find ways to arrange by priority everything I need to do so I can cope with it all.

1. _____ _____

2. _____ _____

3. _____ _____

4. _____ _____

5. _____ _____

6. _____ _____

SEPARATING DISABILITY-RELATED
FROM NON-DISABILITY-RELATED ISSUES

The impact of an illness or disability can be far-reaching indeed. These realities can greatly affect the life-style, goals, needs, and strengths of a person and his or her family. As discussed in Chapter 5, family needs in each of the eight basic areas can become intensified in families with ill or disabled members. However, even though it may be convenient to attribute all of one's problems to an illness or disability or all family problems to the member with the special need, that is rarely, if ever, the true state of affairs. As we noted in Chapter 1, some problems are caused by an illness or disability, and other problems are complicated by it. Still other problems have nothing to do with the special need at all. The ability to separate disability-related from non-disability-related issues is very helpful to the problem-solving process.

The tendency to attribute the cause of family problems to a member's illness or disability can be a dangerous lure *and* trap for families. All of us have certain strengths and limitations. To focus on any one of these as the primary component of our selfhood is incorrect and can limit our ability both to maximize our strengths and to develop in other areas. Furthermore, it can distract from the true source of a problem and, thus, can camouflage a number of useful solutions. In the course of our daily lives, problems are often less the result of a special need per se than of the complex demands of life and the conflicting needs of family members. All families have needs and problems, be they juggling strained finances or coping with the onset of puberty in adolescent children.

For example, it is extremely common for American parents to experience difficulty in "letting go" of their adolescent children. Adolescents experience similar difficulty in letting go of their parents. In the case of an adolescent with a disability or illness, it is not uncommon for parents to focus excessively on the child's special needs and to point to them as the primary cause of the child's delay in leaving home (and hence the reason he or she should remain safe at home!). This situation is reminiscent of that of the Buonomo family in Chapter 1. Rather than Stephanie's blindness causing the problem of transition, it merely intensified a problem that is common to many families—separation. Thus, in order for successful launching to occur, it is important that families reevaluate the true nature of the situation. This type of redefinition can ease the adolescent's efforts to separate from his or her family and grow while increasing the parents' independence from their child. The following case study helps illustrate the pitfalls of an illness or disability focus to problem solving and the benefits of distinguishing problems unrelated to a family member's special needs.

James Washington is 13 years old. He lives with his mother and younger brother Ricky. James has a congenital cleft lip and palate for which he has undergone nine surgical procedures. Despite this extensive surgical repair, James still has some speech problems and cosmetic damage.

James has become particularly conscious of his disability in the past year. Importantly, this self-consciousness corresponds to his growing interest in girls and peer relationships. James believes that because of his speech and appearance, others regard him as "a freak" and reject his friendship. As a result, James has become withdrawn and isolated at school, and he experiences a pervasive depression. In addition, he argues extensively with his mother and brother at home. James accuses his mother of irresponsibly bringing him into this world "maimed" and states that he'd rather be dead than remain so ugly. James fights with his younger brother Ricky, insisting that Ricky is favored and flaunts his good looks. James's mother and brother respond to these accusations by insisting that his appearance is much improved since the latest surgery and that future operations will relieve his problem even more.

Because of his intense unhappiness and increasing conflict at home, Mrs. Washington encouraged James to discuss his feelings with her. However, when these discussions consistently turned into fights, Mrs. Washington insisted that James speak with a counselor. A meeting was arranged, and although reluctant at first, James consented to follow through.

James explained to the counselor that he was ugly and "a jerk" because of his cleft lip and palate and that nobody wanted to spend time with him at school. He cried, saying that at times he hated his disability so much that he wished he was dead. The counselor, attentive to his great unmet needs for acceptance and self-esteem, suggested that he attend a therapy group with other boys his age.

Much to James's surprise, he discovered that the other boys in the group had needs, concerns, and sensitivities similar to his own. Initially, he told the other members that his only problem was his "messed-up face." The boys were interested in the cause of James's facial disfigurement, asked numerous questions, and seemed to sympathize with his problem. As the group progressed and James persisted in focusing solely on his disability, however, the other boys challenged this overriding belief. They said that his appearance was not the only thing they noticed in him and that it was a "cop out" to blame all his troubles on his disability. James was quite taken back at this new perspective and at first tried to defend his belief that his looks were central to his social status. Through the course of the group, James and the other boys engaged in further discussions about making friends, talking to girls, trying to "fit in," and dealing with parents on issues of freedom and responsibility. Gradually, after much work, James began to see that he was not abnormal in his need to fit in or in his difficulty in doing so. He learned that other boys, regardless of their looks, had similar insecurities about socializing and meeting girls. Furthermore, as living testimony to these new insights, James discovered that the other boys in the group had readily accepted him as a member. In fact, they seemed more interested in his ideas and feelings than in his looks.

This experience proved helpful to James in several ways. First, it forced him to examine and appreciate aspects of himself other than his appearance. Second, it helped him attribute less blame and importance to his disability as he learned that it was only as much of a handicap as he made it. Third, once able to gauge the response of others to his disability, James was able to shed some of his disabling beliefs about the hopelessness of his appearance. James was also able to take risks and begin experimenting with social interactions. As a result, James began to reach out more to others at school, improve his social skills, and develop some meaningful friendships. He subsequently became less argumentative at home, as both James and his family began to appreciate the many strengths he possessed. Thus, the Washingtons learned to differentiate issues directly related to James's cleft lip and palate from those that had little to do with the disability itself.

This case study exemplifies how easily an individual and a family can focus attention on a disability even though it may not represent the true nature of a problem. Although James may be aware of certain limitations his disability does pose, these limitations do not have to interfere with his needs for acceptance and friendship. Clearly, appearance is important to most adolescents, but each teenager must learn that other aspects of his or her personality and talents are equally worthy of love and respect. In James's case, by focusing excessively on his disability, this normal process became all the more difficult. Thus, learning to separate disability- and illness-related issues from non-disability- and non-illness-related issues is an invaluable skill from which all families can benefit. Exercise 7D can help you develop this skill.

Exercise 7D

Look back at the list of problem definitions you developed in Exercise 7C. Put a "U" beside each one that you think is unrelated to your family member's illness or disability. For example, a family might decide that a problem defined as obtaining better financial opportunities is not related to illness or disability. Put an "R" beside those problems that you think are primarily caused by the special need; for example, alleviating a family member's depression following a traumatic accident. Third, put a "B" beside those problems that involve issues both related and unrelated to the special need of an ill or disabled family member.

Next, choose *two* of the problems from your list, and see if you can differentiate which aspects of each relate to the special need and which do not. Here are two examples:

Example 1:

Problem definition: Determine vocational choice for an adolescent with paraplegia. **B**

Disability-related issues: 1) physical limitations, 2) accessible location, 3) overcoming potential discrimination

Non-disability-related issues: 1) preferences and goals, 2) self-concept and confidence, 3) fears

Example 2 (from Exercise 7C, Example A):

Problem definition: I need a plan to figure out how to get money for the equipment I need. **B**

Disability-related issues: Need medication, equipment, resources depleted by other disability-related needs

Non-disability-related issues: Economically disadvantaged, anger at system, preference to spend money on other things

1. *Problem definition:* _____
   _____
   _____

   Disability-related issues: _____
   _____
   _____

   Non-disability-related issues: _____
   _____
   _____

(continued)

Exercise 7D
(continued)

2. *Problem definition:* _____
   _____
   _____

   Disability-related issues: _____
   _____
   _____

   Non-disability-related issues: _____
   _____
   _____

HOW TO COPE WITH "UNSOLVABLE" PROBLEMS: DEFINING AREAS YOU CAN CONTROL

Clearly, not all life circumstances are under our direct control. Crime, natural disaster, discrimination, and the onset of a disability or illness are but a few examples of situations we cannot choose to face or avoid. Fortunately, how we respond to these "slings and arrows" of life is under our direct control. We *can* choose the manner in which we respond to a crisis and thus mitigate its impact upon us. For example, although we cannot control other people's behavior, we can choose how we wish to respond to their actions. Thus, a person with leukemia whose chemotherapy has caused baldness can respond to the stares of strangers with a scowl, a smile, or indifference. Similarly, an individual who determines that she is being given the runaround by a service system can choose to respond with anger, resignation, or assertiveness. Despite the many obstacles we face in life, it is liberating to realize that, yes, we do have control over how we cope.

Similar to separating illness- or disability-related from non-illness or non-disability-related issues, differentiating between circumstances we can and cannot control is invaluable to effective problem solving. Suppose, for example, that a problem has been defined as diabetes, paralysis, or dyslexia. This type of definition may pose an "unsolvable" problem. However, if these same problems were defined in terms of areas one can influence, problem solving becomes feasible and productive. Thus, reframing diabetes in terms of manageable elements, such as: 1) controlling blood sugar levels, 2) arranging for frequent meals, 3) adapting to new activity levels, or 4) dealing with feelings about having a chronic illness, can add greatly to one's control over one's life. Similarly, redefining the problem of paralysis in terms of transportation problems, loss of self-esteem, or feelings of despair creates a starting place for effecting change and becoming unstuck from seemingly unsolvable dilemmas. Exercise 7E provides you with an opportunity to reframe problems that you may have previously considered unsolvable into controllable, manageable components.

SELECTING A PROBLEM TO ADDRESS

With the many needs we encounter daily and the many unmet needs that may go unidentified over time, how can we know where to begin

---

Exercise 7E

List three problems that have recently or in the past seemed unsolvable. Spend a few minutes thinking of aspects of each problem that you can control, manage, and change. Do these aspects seem easier to target for resolution than the problems you first listed?

"Unsolvable" Problems	Controllable Aspects
1.	a.
	b.
	c.
	d.
2.	a.
	b.
	c.
	d.
3.	a.
	b.
	c.
	d.

---

addressing them? Selecting one of several problems to address can be a challenge in and of itself. Thus, knowing your priorities can be the first step toward determining which of two or more needs to address first.

Similar to the way in which individual families emphasize needs to varying degrees, families rely on their priorities in their decisions to give certain needs more attention than others. For example, in particularly health-conscious families, needs related to members' safety, nutrition, medical care, and fitness are liable to receive the utmost attention. These priorities might outweigh, for example, recreational or educational needs and are attended to first. In a family where one member is about to lose her job and another is on the verge of an emotional breakdown, family members may choose to work on the emotional issue before the financial one. Thus, each family's priorities determine its choice of problem to address.

It is important to point out here that priorities are not necessarily equated with values. For example, although a family might value education more than money in the grand scheme of things, if finances are a particular problem, monetary issues may take on a higher priority than usual. That is, although a financial crisis might not wait, buying a set of encyclopedias or choosing a college may be less urgent. Thus, priorities in a family may change over time, depending on resources and the varied demands of different life-cycle stages.

Families have a variety of criteria by which they informally choose which problems to address before others. The following criteria are used by some families in problem selection:

1. Involves health and security of members
2. Is easy to resolve
3. Affects many people
4. Has long-range implications
5. Involves the independence of family members
6. Involves finances
7. Involves educational advancement
8. Is putting a stress on more than one family need

This partial list provides room for you to include the criteria your own family considers important. Exercise 7F will help your family identify its priorities in selecting a problem to address.

Obviously, the process of deciding on a problem to address is not always complicated. More often than not, your family may have agreed automatically to work together on some problem without pausing to think why you were choosing one issue over another. Some of the problems you listed in this chapter may already be solved; perhaps all it took was getting a concern out in the open. Or perhaps you have one problem that is *so* pressing that comparing it to others seems a bit silly. Nonetheless, we have suggested that you do this step-by-step exercise for several important reasons. First, we wanted you to clarify and clearly state the criteria you were probably already using unconsciously. Second, people in your family whose problems

---

Exercise 7F

Look back at the six case studies in Chapter 1 and choose one family. Pretend that this family has asked yours to tell them which of their many problems they need to work on first. Either individually or as a group, think of criteria you deem important for selecting a problem to address.

List them briefly:

1. _____ _____
2. _____ _____
3. _____ _____
4. _____ _____
5. _____ _____
6. _____ _____
7. _____ _____
8. _____ _____
9. _____ _____
10. _____ _____

Talk over your criteria as a family, and try to reach agreement on the five most important criteria. Put a "1" through "5" beside each one of these, in order of importance.

Now, look at the problem definitions for your own family in Exercise 7C, and try to use the criteria you just listed to select one problem to address. Briefly state each problem definition in the spaces on the left-hand side of the worksheet on the next page. Then, think whether your first problem meets criterion number 1; if it does, put a check ($\sqrt{}$) in the box. Do the same with criteria numbers 2–5. Continue in this way until you have rated all your problem definitions. Talk over your answers with each other. Can you reach agreement on a problem to solve first? (If you need more room, do this exercise on a separate sheet.)

(continued)

Exercise 7F
(continued)

Problems	Criteria				
	1	2	3	4	5
1. _____	☐	☐	☐	☐	☐
2. _____	☐	☐	☐	☐	☐
3. _____	☐	☐	☐	☐	☐
4. _____	☐	☐	☐	☐	☐
5. _____	☐	☐	☐	☐	☐
6. _____	☐	☐	☐	☐	☐

have been temporarily set aside can understand why and thus not feel their problems are being neglected (as long as you have all agreed to come back to those later!). Third, many family problems are inter-related. By separating them into different problems and carefully deciding which to address first, you may have the key to the other problem. It's very much like finding the end of a tangled length of string that you want to untangle and roll into a smooth ball—first you must know where to start. In the next chapter we discuss how families can best proceed in devising solutions to well-defined problems.

CHAPTER

8

Brainstorming

Once you are aware of the many resources available to your family, you can begin thinking about different alternatives for solving problems and satisfying needs. Given the resources you have identified within your family, you social support network, and your community, you may be amazed at the number of possible solutions that come to mind.

The process of generating alternatives to solve a particular problem is called brainstorming. For example, if you had only 15 minutes to eat dinner before making an 8:00 P.M. movie, you might quickly and spontaneously brainstorm a number of alternatives:

1. Pick up a fast hamburger to eat on the way.
2. Wait until after the movie to eat.
3. Eat popcorn in the movie to tide you over until a late dinner.
4. Enjoy a leisurely dinner and postpone the movie.
5. Skip dinner altogether.
6. Smuggle some food into the theatre to eat during the movie.

Brainstorming is a process we use everyday in both casual and complex situations. It is a process by which we generate practical options to clearcut problems, as well as to seemingly unsolvable dilemmas. Although the process of problem solving is oriented toward accomplishing change and resolution as efficiently as possible, it is also a technique to manage and alleviate long-range problems. The following case example illustrates the valuable use of the brainstorming process in dealing with a seemingly elusive and unsolvable problem: the loss of one's future hopes and dreams.

The Delaney family has grappled for years with the trauma and turmoil surrounding the onset of Michael's symptoms of paranoid schizophrenia. Currently 23 years old, Michael has endured the chaos of his illness for 8 years. His parents, Sam and Laura, have traveled with Michael the long road of violent behavioral problems, misdiagnoses, troubles with the police, suicide attempts, school expulsions, and medication side effects. From institution to home and back again, the Delaneys have suffered the chaos of living with a chronic mental illness.

Before developing symptoms of schizophrenia, Michael had taken pleasure and his parents had shown pride in his close friendships and special talents. A particularly talented guitarist, Michael had been active in a number of musical groups and eventually hoped to record some of his songs.

Gradually, however, Michael's dreams and behavior began to deteriorate. After he had been missing for 5 days, Michael reappeared and began to exhibit clear symptoms of schizophrenia. For the next 5 years, he and his family sought every means and every hope of recovery. Only recently did Sam and Laura accept the fact of Michael's chronic illness. He is now spending his time between the state hospital and a half-way house, and Sam and Laura have begun to pick up the pieces of their disrupted lives and shattered dreams.

Every day, each of the Delaneys deals with his or her own sense of ruined aspirations and lost hope. The feeling of forever is what bears so heavily on each of them. For Sam and Laura, the knowledge of Michael's wasted talents and grim prognosis necessitates that they reevaluate their own goals and reset their sights based on the harsh realities they have confronted. They have defined their most salient problem—their loss of hopes and dreams—and targeted it for resolution.

The Delaneys sought the help of a clinical psychologist with whom they had previously established a strong working alliance. There, in the safety of her private office, the Delaneys and the psychologist brainstormed alternative ways of coping with their lost hope. These options ranged from the sublime (praying to God for a miracle) to the seemingly ridiculous (moving to Tahiti forever). Yet, among these varied ideas, the Delaneys and the therapist were able to brainstorm a number of ways to cope with the seemingly unsolvable. These included: 1) redefining their own goals, separate from those they held for Michael; 2) taking some time out to deal with the loss before actively making changes; 3) enlisting the support and love of friends and family; 4) reevaluating their hopes for Michael to put them on a more realistic scale; 5) stopping blaming themselves and focusing more on taking care of their own needs; 6) finding purpose and meaning in helping other people with similar life circumstances; 7) working through their feelings by sharing with each other, as well as with other individuals; 8) stopping denying the reality and future reality of Michael's illness and focusing on acceptance; 9) stopping assuming responsibilities for Michael's choices, and 10) channeling some of their feelings of anger and helplessness into political advocacy programs for individuals with emotional disabilities. Thus, after some concerted effort, the Delaneys had accomplished a crucial step in the problem-solving process: generating a number of alternatives for dealing with the defined problem. From these options, they were able to begin evaluating each alternative before choosing a plan of action.

This case example illustrates the value of brainstorming in coping with problems. Without the willingness to pause and solicit alternative solutions from yourself and others, to cooperate and share ideas, it is difficult to proceed effectively toward resolving family problems. The following discussion helps clarify specific elements of the brainstorming process as it can be applied to your own family problems.

THE BRAINSTORMING PROCESS

Brainstorming in a group, such as a family, adds a valuable dimension to the process. With more people participating, it is likely that more alternatives will be generated. The key to successful brainstorming is quantity, not necessarily quality. Thus, it is important that as many family members as possible participate in the brainstorming process. You may also want to include a close friend or someone else in your support system, even if long distance communication is necessary. Of course, determining which members to involve is an individual decision that varies from problem to problem and family to family. For example, the people who are affected by the problem, those who are interested in participating, resource persons who are likely to have helpful ideas, and those who can meet the practical requirements of attending discussion sessions or communicating by long distance differ for every family and every problem. Families may further need to consider the age at which children should be encouraged to participate, the manner in which a member with communication difficulties can most fully contribute, and who may be affected by the solution. These questions may elicit different viewpoints among family members and require communication and negotiation skills in order to arrive at a decision.

Exercise 8A is designed to help your family begin exploring issues in a structured way concerning who should be involved in brainstorming for a particular problem. Although such an activity may seem a bit tedious and cumbersome, we suggest it to help you systematically think through the reasons for involving appropriate persons in the brainstorming process. Sometimes we tend to inappropriately exclude some family members, friends, or professionals and to include others merely because "that's the way we have always done it." Because every problem is different, the people who can help think of possible alternatives also vary. Although it is up to your family to determine whom to include in the brainstorming process, it is helpful to keep in mind the value of added input.

In order to generate a large number of alternatives, strive to encourage all brainstorming participants to suggest spontaneous ideas without evaluating either the merits or disadvantages of the idea (that comes later). Censoring ideas is a pitfall to be avoided. Overcoming our tendency to censor our own and others' thoughts enables us to break out of established patterns of thinking and to generate innovative ideas. Censoring, or not revealing ideas judged to be unworthy of consideration, is a process we engage in both privately and publicly. Consider the following case:

Peter, a young man with cerebral palsy who did not have the use of his hands or arms, felt highly dependent on others to assist him with many of his everyday needs (e.g., eating, brushing his teeth). Although Peter was exceptionally dexterous with his feet, he found it difficult to suggest using his feet for many of these activities. He feared that others would find this shocking or embarrassing. Fortunately, he finally stopped censoring this "crazy" idea and posed it as an alternative to his family. At first, they were unaccustomed to seeing someone eat with his feet, but they soon accepted this alterna-

Exercise 8A

Using one problem identified in Chapter 7, work through the following three steps in order to determine whom to involve in the brainstorming process.

Step 1: List your family members and any possible friends, community people, or professionals who may be helpful in solving this problem. You may want to refer to your inventory of social and professional support in Chapter 3 (Exercise 3A).

1.   9.
2.   10.
3.   11.
4.   12.
5.   13.
6.   14.
7.   15.
8.   16.

Step 2: Which issues are important to consider concerning whom to involve in decision making? We have provided a few, but add your own to the list. Determine whether each potential participant meets each of the criteria on your list.

1. Affected by problem?
2. Wants to participate?
3. Has expertise?
4. Provides different perspective?
5. Creative?
6. _____
7. _____
8. _____
9. _____
10. _____
11. _____
12. _____

Step 3: Briefly list whom you decided to involve and why. If someone you want to include has not met many of the criteria, explain why you still want to involve him or her (e.g., his opinion is important to us; she is caring and honest; he is willing to contribute).

tive as an excellent opportunity for increasing Peter's independence, as well as the rest of the family's.

Peter and his family have continued to experiment with new ideas and have enjoyed increased freedom and autonomy as a result. As one might expect from so creative and assertive an individual, Peter is now highly independent and successful. He continues to utilize his foot coordination for a number of activities ranging from typing his own memos to lighting matches.

Thus, in Peter's case, a viable and liberating alternative might have been ignored because its originator feared public rebuke and chose to censor it. Similarly, Peter's family could have prematurely rejected his idea, criticizing his behavior on the basis of what they were accustomed to observing in others. Fortunately, both Peter and his family were open to this, as well as other, innovative ideas. This openness increased their freedom as individuals within the family.

Often, we have the tendency to judge our own or others' ideas before they have been given due consideration. For example, we might consider an idea silly or impractical and fail to suggest it to others. Or we might react to another's suggestion with criticism, ridicule, argument, or other forms of immediate evaluation. These tendencies are counterproductive in brainstorming because they hinder the open expression of spontaneous ideas. At a later point, of course, it is appropriate and, indeed, imperative to evaluate the usefulness of each alternative. During brainstorming, however, the goal is to encourage a quantity of ideas in an open and nonjudgmental atmosphere. The ability to generate a large number of ideas can be accomplished through practice, risk taking, and some encouragement.

Ideally, a given brainstorming session should include **all** the people you want to participate in solving a problem. This is how brainstorming works best. One person may toss out an idea, which triggers a thought in another person, and so forth. The give-and-take of the group generally yields more ideas than having each person individually think of alternatives and then bring them to the group. We recognize, however, that getting everybody together at one time to brainstorm about a family problem may not always be possible. We hope you will try out a variety of approaches to see what works best for your family. For example, you might brainstorm in groups of three or four on some occasions. Or after brainstorming in a group that includes most of the people who are participating, you might talk to those who couldn't be there by phone or in person and gain their input. One family we know conducted their brainstorming sessions during commercials as they watched TV. They made a game of seeing how many ideas they could produce during each break. The point is this: Do what is comfortable for *you*.

To practice expressing ideas and accepting those of others, try Exercise 8B with as many of your family members as you can gather.

When you have a feel for the brainstorming process, it's time to try it out on a problem of your own. Exercise 8C is designed to guide you through the process.

Once you have gone through a brainstorming session with your family, stop and think about your experience. In particular, consider the different roles each participant played. Who led the discussion? Did everyone participate? Who participated the least? Who participated the most? Was everyone's behavior typical of most family interactions? Did participants feel that their ideas were met with encouragement and approval? Talk these questions over with your family. It might be useful for you to repeat Exercise 8C, with each person assuming a *different* role than he or she took in the first session

---

Exercise 8B

Consider the following case study:

> Matt and Nina Galanto have been married for 5 years. Since Matt suffered a spinal cord injury 1 year after their marriage, both have had to make a number of adjustments. Nina has taken on much of the financial responsibility, working as a typist, while Matt is employed part-time as a math tutor.
>
> Matt has tried to adjust to a greater degree of dependence on Nina than he finds comfortable. Particularly troubling to Matt is his wife's constant involvement in many of his personal care needs. On the one hand, Matt feels that he needs help bathing, dressing, and so forth, and appreciates Nina's help. Yet, on the other hand, he has come to resent his dependence and finds her help intrusive and embarrassing. Similarly, although Nina feels responsible for helping Matt, she is finding that the physical strain and constant tension are taking their toll on her as well. As a result, Matt and Nina have defined a problem: Matt and Nina need greater independence from each other, primarily in terms of Matt's personal care needs.

What alternatives might the Galantos consider to resolve their current problem? As a family, generate as many alternatives as possible for the Galantos' situation. Write them down on a separate piece of paper. Try to make sure each participant contributes at least one idea. (*Note:* If you feel you don't have enough facts about this family to generate many solutions, invent the facts! The idea of this exercise is for your family to practice being as creative as possible.)

Exercise 8C

Convene as many of the brainstorming participants you identified in
Exercise 8A as possible. Choose a current family problem—for example
one identified in a previous exercise—and begin to brainstorm alternative
means of satisfying that need. Everyone involved should be encouraged to
contribute ideas. Be careful not to censor your own or other members'
ideas or to evaluate their suggestions in any way. In other words, emphasize creativity; suggest seemingly unusual ideas. Children can be encouraged to contribute their ideas particularly well in a nonjudgmental and
open brainstorming session. Their imagination and lack of inhibitions
may spark many new ideas with a little added encouragement and reinforcement. Record a list of all the alternatives generated by your family on
a separate sheet of paper. (Be sure to save it for use in the exercises in the
next chapter.) Talk to anyone who was unable to attend the brainstorming
session, and add their ideas to your list.

(use the same problem or a different one, if you like). For example,
assign a new person to take the most active role and another to take
the least active role. One person might be given the specific job of
helping everyone contribute. Experiment. Brainstorming should be
approached in a flexible way that fits your own particular family style.

The main goals of brainstorming can be summarized in three
key points. First, it is important to include as many participants as
possible, especially those who are affected by the problem. Second,
quantity is the secret to successful brainstorming. Be creative, spontaneous, and open to exchanging ideas in a nonjudgmental and non-
self-conscious manner. Finally, be aware of your common patterns of
interaction. Perhaps there is an important voice that is heard far too
infrequently and other voices that tend to dominate. Brainstorming is
the starting point for building a spirit of family cooperation and
communication—the foundation of successful problem solving.

CHAPTER

9

Evaluating and
Choosing Alternatives

Once a number of alternative solutions have been brainstormed, it is time to evaluate their potential usefulness. Obviously, not every problem is so complicated as to require exhaustive evaluation. Perhaps just expressing an unmet need or defining a problem, as you did in Chapter 7, is enough to resolve it.

Yet, even when solutions are simple or alternatives are obvious, it is important to stop and think about the potential consequences of the actions you want to take. There are also times when the answers are not so simple or the best alternative not so clearly apparent. We are suggesting, therefore, a framework for evaluating alternatives that you either can work through quickly or, depending on the circumstances, study in a more detailed fashion. This framework involves four basic steps.

The first evaluation step is to narrow down the large number of spontaneous alternatives generated by your family to those alternatives requiring cooperation and negotiation among family members. The second step involves family discussion and the use of "thumbs up" or "thumbs down" ratings of each alternative requiring cooperation and negotiation. This process further excludes weak alternatives and clarifies the positive elements of the remaining alternatives. Step 3 is to evaluate these positive alternatives with respect to your family's special needs, values, and concerns. This entails the use of specific criteria. These criteria can help clarify the most fruitful course of action and, thus, the most productive alternatives. Finally, once you have examined your options in light of important criteria, step 4 is to decide on a course of action.

These steps will become easier to follow with the help of more detailed explanations and case examples provided throughout this chapter. For now, it is important to note that the evaluation and choice of alternatives rely heavily on your use of the communication and negotiation skills described in Chapter 6.

Suppose that your family has arrived at a long list of varied solutions to a problem. In addition to following the four evaluation steps just outlined, what can your family do throughout this process to ensure that the best alternative is adopted as the solution? A number of suggestions can help minimize problems that may occur further down the road, such as during the actual implementation of your chosen solution. First and foremost, it is important for each family member to be actively involved. Each member needs to take responsibility for evaluating the impact of an alternative on his or her own well-being. This expression of one's personal stake in a particular alternative adds a great deal to the evaluation process as it enables family members to consider the needs of everyone else as well. One young woman with degenerative arthritis told us:

> I knew that if I went into the hospital for intensive treatment, my family would be relieved of a big burden. They wouldn't have to turn me over in the middle of the night, or hear me cry. I hated the idea myself, but thought it would be best to just keep my mouth shut.

By failing to express herself, this woman missed an opportunity to avoid an unpleasant alternative and allow other members to express their feelings regarding hospitalization. It is quite possible that other alternatives (e.g., home care, home physical therapy, outpatient treatment) could have been instituted in such a way that all family members' needs would have been met more fully. It may be helpful to keep in mind here that everyone affects everyone else in a family. Thus, voicing your opinion of an alternative is as much a responsibility as it is a right.

In this vein, children and family members with intellectual and physical disabilities should be encouraged to participate as fully as possible. Thus, the use of a communication board or a computer by a family member having cerebral palsy, specific questions directed to children, and a good deal of support and encouragement of a family member with mental retardation can go a long way toward validating their importance within the family. These individuals' input can be crucial to the effective evaluation of alternatives.

Finally, you may want to continue involving any friends or professionals whom you included in the brainstorming process. During your brainstorming session, you may have produced some ideas that involved other people who were not initially included. If so, you might consider expanding your problem-solving circle to include them or at least check whether or not they are willing to help. There is no formula for precisely whom to include, except that you should do what is most comfortable for your own family. These considerations should guide your family's efforts through each step of the evaluation process.

STEP 1: COOPERATION AND NEGOTIATION RESOLVES PROBLEMS

The first step in the evaluation process involves assigning alternatives to one of three general categories:

1. Alternatives that avoid the problem
2. Alternatives demanding that only one person change
3. Alternatives involving cooperation and negotiation among family members

In order to understand how these three categories enter into problem solving, consider the following example:

Mr. and Mrs. Singer are a young couple. For the past 5 months, Mr. Singer has been disabled by severe lower back pain, the cause of which is as yet unknown. During these 5 months, the Singers have been unable to engage in their normal pattern of sexual relations. Mrs. Singer is especially dissatisfied with their infrequent sexual contact and would like to determine some alternatives for meeting both her and her husband's sexual needs. Mr. Singer is also frustrated and would like to resolve their current difficulties. Consider the following possible alternatives from each of the three categories listed above:

Alternatives that avoid the problem:

1. *Put the issue on hold and see how things progress.*
2. *Have Mrs. Singer spend more time with friends.*
3. *Spend more time together enjoying music and cards.*
4. *Find a better physician for Mr. Singer.*
5. *Accept the situation until Mr. Singer has fully recovered.*

These alternatives do not address the sexual needs that the Singers have targeted for resolution in their problem statement. Instead, they successfully avoid the issue, focusing on safe yet unproductive "solutions." Thus, alternatives that can be determined to fall into the category of avoiding the problem are best reworked or discarded altogether.

Alternatives demanding that only one person change:

1. *Have Mr. Singer see a counselor.*
2. *Have Mrs. Singer satisfy her sexual needs without Mr. Singer.*
3. *Have Mr. Singer explore potential variations to their normal sex life.*
4. *Have Mrs. Singer attempt new ways of arousing Mr. Singer.*

Again, these alternatives are unlikely to resolve the Singers' current needs. By placing responsibility only on one partner's shoulders, the other is left exempt from active participation and responsibility. Similarly, one partner's individual needs are left unheard. Thus, if failure results, one partner is often blamed or scapegoated. The Singers will obtain their best opportunity for success by employing alternatives that involve mutual cooperation and negotiation. As a rule, alternatives that demand that only one person change should be rejected.

Alternatives that involve cooperation and negotiation:

1. *Have the Singers seek sexual counseling together.*
2. *Have the Singers experiment with new forms of physical intimacy that do not require Mr. Singer to "perform" sexually.*
3. *Increase the time spent touching and cuddling to fulfill some affectional needs.*

4. *Have open communication about sexual needs and desires.*

5. *Obtain literature on sexual options and discuss them together.*

These alternatives require that the Singers engage in an ongoing process of cooperation and negotiation. That is, by considering their own and each other's needs in a spirit of joint endeavor, the Singers can work together to overcome their current difficulties and develop a more satisfying sex life. The goal, then, in evaluating alternatives is to determine those alternatives that involve cooperation and negotiation. Alternatives that fall into one or both of the first two categories should be reformulated or rejected altogether. Consider the following situation:

Mary and Tom Jones have been married for 3 years. Both have been hearing-impaired since birth. For the past year, they have seriously considered having a baby and have carefully worked through many of the issues that initially concerned them. One issue remains a central obstacle to their ability to feel prepared and confident to start a family: They both work full-time, and neither wants to sacrifice a career nor much-needed family income. Having identified this issue, they brainstorm the following list of alternative solutions:

1. *Do not ever have a baby.*

2. *Have a baby, and then take things as they come.*

3. *Arrange for Mary to quit her job.*

4. *Arrange for Mary to take a 1-year leave of absence and for Tom to work overtime.*

5. *Arrange for Tom to quit his job.*

6. *Arrange for Tom and Mary both to take on half-time work.*

7. *Arrange for Tom and Mary to alternate a 1-year leave of absence.*

8. *Take out a loan, and arrange for child care.*

9. *Take out a loan, and have Tom and/or Mary reduce their work times.*

10. *Arrange for extended family members or neighbors to help with the child care responsibilities.*

As Table 9.1. illustrates, these 10 alternatives can be easily assigned into one or more of the three categories described above. This

Table 9.1. Assigning alternatives to categories

Alternatives	Categories			Why statements
	Avoids problems	Demands that only one change	Cooperation and negotiation	
1. Never have a baby			X	Both of us need to discuss this possibility further and negotiate a mutually agreeable decision.
2. Play it by ear	X			Putting off making plans will not alleviate the financial and career decisions identified as issues.
3. Mary quits job	X	X		Requires that only Mary change and fails to address the financial issues involved with the loss of income.
4. Mary takes leave, Tom works overtime			X	Requires that both of us compromise and both take responsibility for fulfilling our child care and financial needs.
5. Tom quits job	X	X		Requires that only Tom change and poses a financial problem already identified.
6. Tom and Mary work 50%			X	Requires that both of us make career sacrifices and cooperate with child care and financial responsibilities.
7. Tom and Mary alternate leaves of absence			X	Involves a mutual arrangement of work time so we both retain careers yet fulfill child care needs.
8. Take out loan plus child care			X	Requires a mutual financial investment in both a loan and in child care payments.

(continued)

Table 9.1. *(continued)*

Alternatives	Categories			Why statements
	Avoids problems	Demands that only one change	Cooperation and negotiation	
9. Take out loan, plus both reduce worktime			X	Involves a mutual financial commitment plus cooperation in terms of work scheduling.
10. Solicit child care help from social support system			X	Enables both of us to continue working while cooperatively arranging help from family and friends.

process enables Tom and Mary to rule out clearly ineffective alternatives, because only those involving cooperation and negotiation are appropriate for family problem solving. A large range of options are narrowed down to fewer yet better ones that are geared toward success. Table 9.1. reveals that Tom and Mary have many viable alternatives. The need to reformulate or reject alternatives is clarified by employing a "why" statement with each decision. Thus, Mary might say, "I do not want to quit my job. We will not make enough money and I will be entirely responsible for taking care of the baby during the day." This type of clarifying communication makes the alternative's shortcomings apparent to everyone involved and invites suggestions for improvement or rejection. During open discussions of this type, differences of opinion often arise. Such differences can provide valuable insight into the issue at hand, especially when family members conscientiously use good communication skills. Exercise 9A is designed to help your family do the first step of evaluating alternatives. A blank worksheet that looks like Table 9.1 by Tom and Mary is provided at the end of this book (along with all the other exercises) to help you list your family's alternatives.

STEP 2:   TO KEEP OR NOT TO KEEP—RATING ALTERNATIVES

Once the alternatives are narrowed down to those that involve cooperation and negotiation among family members, you are ready to

---

Exercise 9A

Using the list obtained from your brainstorming exercise in Chapter 8, gather the family together for an evaluation session. If this is not convenient, each person could do this exercise separately and compare results later. Worksheet 9A, which is similar to Table 9.1 in which Mary and Tom Jones evaluated their alternatives, is blank. Put your own problem statement (from Chapter 7) at the top of the page and brief descriptions of each of your brainstormed alternatives down the side. If you are doing this exercise as a group, have one member read each alternative, and then decide together to which category it belongs. Record your answers in the table. Encourage everyone in the family to participate, and include a "why" statement along with each decision. Practice accepting others' opinions as helpful input, avoiding criticism or argument. When differences of opinion do arise, use the negotiation and communication skills you have acquired to resolve them.

---

begin selecting alternatives to put into action. At this point, it is vital that all family members involved in the problem-solving process participate and take responsibility for discussing the personal and familial implications of each alternative solution. The best way to accomplish this type of communication and interchange of ideas is by arranging a common meeting time. Then, by taking turns, each member can express his or her feelings and thoughts about each potential alternative, accompanied by a "thumbs up" or "thumbs down" opinion. Here again, it is crucial to fully include the family member with an illness or disability. If this member is simply unable to participate due to absence or severe illness, family members can make an effort to consider this person's perspective as best as possible. An effective solution is best ensured by considering the perspectives and feelings of all family members.

After each member has given an opinion and explained why each alternative was rated positively or negatively, these ratings can be tallied and the majority opinion adopted. Thus, if three members rate an alternative "plus," and two rate it "minus," the alternative should not yet be rejected. Ties can either be negotiated to a reject or retain decision after some additional discussion or simply retained until all the positive alternatives are evaluated further. As you can see, evaluating, and choosing, alternatives is largely a process of elimination. The family discerns problems in the faulty alternatives and discards them, thereby clarifying the good options still available. The following case study illustrates this step in the evaluation process.

Mark Chang is a 20-year-old adolescent who has been diagnosed as manic-depressive. He lives at home with his parents and an older sister Sharon. Despite extensive psychiatric consultations and medication reviews, Mark's behavior is highly unpredictable. From day to day, he swings between periods of agitation and destructiveness, and severe depression and suicidality. On various occasions, Mark has broken windows in the house, slashed the furniture with a kitchen knife, and attempted suicide by both overdosing and slashing his wrists. As a result, it is imperative that someone be available to Mark at all times. Although hospitalization has been required on several occasions, all the Changs prefer that Mark remain at home if at all possible.

The Changs identified a problem in the family when Mrs. Chang expressed her unhappiness and feelings of stress over her enormous responsibility for interacting alone with Mark during weekdays. Mr. Chang, who works as a schoolteacher during the day, cannot be home to help Mrs. Chang with Mark. Despite her other commitments, Sharon, a junior college student, has expressed a desire to help. The Changs held a brainstorming session and composed the following list of alternatives:

1. *Have Mrs. Chang continue her involvement with Mark during the day.*
2. *Have Sharon arrange her schedule so that she can help Mrs. Chang during the day.*
3. *Have Mr. Chang ask for time off from work.*
4. *Ignore Mark's behavior and have everyone go about their own business during the day.*
5. *Encourage Mark to agree to hospitalization immediately.*
6. *Accept Gramma's and Grampa's offer to help out part-time.*
7. *Hire someone to stay with Mark part-time.*
8. *Continue treatment attempts to control Mark's depression and destructive behavior.*
9. *Try any of the above alternatives, but consider hospitalization after one month if the situation does not improve.*
10. *Develop a structured program whereby Mark can be involved in productive activities during the day.*

After excluding alternative 1 because it avoided the problem, and postponing alternative 5 within alternative 9, the Changs began the process of selecting one solution from their list. Each family member (including Mark) took a turn stating what they felt would happen if each alternative was tried. They then gave it either a plus or a minus rating, as indicated in Table 9.2. For example, the Changs first discussed accepting Sharon's help. She stated that although it was stressful for her to interact with her brother and difficult for her to take time away from her other commitments, it was extremely important for her to be helpful to her brother. She gave the alternative a plus rating. Mr. Chang felt that Sharon could be helpful in Mark's care, but he felt hesitant to burden her with such responsibility. He felt that the decision to keep Mark outside the hospital had been largely made by him and his wife and that it was unfair to impose such responsibility on Sharon. He gave the alternative a minus rating. Mrs. Chang sympathized with both points of view. However, she felt that a compromise could be reached if Sharon's help was employed as part *of the solution (e.g., one morning or afternoon each week). She gave the alternative a plus rating based on the requirement that it would not be used as an exclusive solution. Mark reiterated his desire to remain outside the hospital and stated that he did not care how he achieved these ends. After being encouraged to state his feelings about Sharon's participation in his care, he said that is was okay with him.*

The Changs continued this discussion until all the alternatives had been evaluated and rated. The alternatives with three or more plus ratings (i.e., a majority) were: 1) enlisting Sharon's daytime help, 2) having Mr. Chang bring as much of his work home as possible in order to increase his at-home time, 3) accepting help from grand-parents, 4) hiring someone to work with Mark one afternoon per week, 5) continuing treatment efforts, 6) developing a structured program of productive activities, and 7) reconsidering hospitalization in one month. The Changs had generated seven viable alternatives for dealing with the stress and demands of Mark's behavior. They were then faced with the task of choosing one or more of these alternatives to put into a plan of action.

To summarize the process of evaluation the Changs have used so far, they 1) reduced their list of alternatives to those requiring cooperation and negotiation, 2) thought about the possible outcomes of each of the remaining alternatives, and 3) individually gave each alternative a plus or minus rating. You have already accomplished the first step of this process in regard to your own family's problem in Exercise 9A. Exercise 9B will guide you in taking the next two steps. A blank worksheet that looks like Table 9.2 that the Chang family filled out is provided at the end of this book (along with all the other exercises) to help you list your family's alternatives.

STEP 3: USING PERSONAL CRITERIA TO CHOOSE THE BEST ALTERNATIVE

In step 3, your family generates criteria to evaluate alternatives based on personal values and priorities. This is a similar process to the one you used in Chapter 7 when you decided which problem to address based on your own criteria. The criteria you use to evaluate alternatives may or may not be the same as those you used to choose a problem. In this case, try to imagine what you would like the results of an alternative to be if it was a perfect solution to your problem. For example, a family placing a great deal of emphasis on independence might list "enhances independence of family members" as one criterion. If the same family is limited in both time and money, it might list "inexpensive" and "takes very little time to do" as two additional criteria. Think back over your family's values (Chapter 2) and needs (Chapter 5) before generating criteria of your own.

Returning to the Chang family, the Changs listed a number of positive results of an *ideal* solution to their problem. According to the Changs, a perfect solution would:

—promote long-term progress
—increase family members' independence
—alleviate stress quickly
—promote health and security
—further intellectual and personal growth
—increase social contact and rewards
—solve additional problems
—not create additional problems
—be easy to carry out
—be enjoyable
—be economical

In Table 9.3., you can see how the Changs listed these criteria down the side of the page. Across the top, they listed each of the alternatives that received a plus rating in Step 2 of their evaluation.

Next, as a family, the Changs thought about which of the criteria would be met by each alternative. For instance, alternative 1

Table 9.2. Evaluating alternatives: The Chang family

Alternatives	Possible outcomes	Family member ratings	Overall ratings
1. Mrs. Chang watches Mark	Rejected: Requires only Mrs. C. change		Minus
2. Sharon helps	a) Reduces strain on Mrs. C. but cuts into Sharon's other activities	Sharon: plus Mrs. C.: plus	Plus
	b) Beneficial to Sharon and Mark's relationship	Mr. C.: minus Mark: plus	
3. Mr. C. requests time off from work	a) Considered impossible given it is mid-semester	Sharon: plus Mrs. C.: plus	Plus
	b) Suggested that Mr. C. could bring as much work home as possible in order to increase at-home time	Mr. C.: plus Mark: minus	
	c) Will alleviate some of other family members' responsibility, and improve father-son relationship		
	d) May initially increase conflict between Mr. C. and Mark		
4. Ignore Mark's behavior	Rejected: Avoids problem		Minus
5. Hospitalize Mark	Reformulated: see Alternative 9 (Avoids problem)		Reformulate
6. Have grandparents help	a) Will alleviate pressure on everyone	Sharon: plus Mrs. C.: plus	Plus
	b) Grandparents have expressed desire to be involved, so should prove a positive alternative for everyone	Mrs. C.: plus Mark: plus	
7. Hire part-time help to spend constructive time with Mark	a) Will alleviate pressure on everyone	Sharon: plus	Plus
	b) Will not strain finances greatly	Mrs. C.: plus	
	c) Will expand Mark's social contact	Mr. C.: plus Mark: plus	
8. Continue treatment	Deemed necessary by everyone	Unanimous plus ratings	Plus
9. Consider hospital in 1 month if no change	Will give timeline to efforts	All but Mark: plus ratings	Plus
10. Plan a structured program	Will enhance Mark's esteem	Unanimous plus ratings	Plus

(Sharon helps out) would alleviate stress quickly, increase social contact for Mark, be easy to carry out, and economical. The Changs put an "X" in the appropriate box beside each criterion that would be met and put a "4" at the bottom. In other words, a total of four criteria would be met by alternative 1. The rest of the alternatives were evaluated in the same manner.

It may be that the problem your family has chosen or the solutions you brainstormed are easier to evaluate than the alternatives the Changs generated. You may have already reached a decision on the best course of action to take. If so, fine. If not *or* if you would like to practice developing and using criteria for choosing alternatives, we

Exercise 9B

Worksheet 9B is a worksheet similar to the one used by the Changs. List those alternatives from Exercise 9A that involve cooperation and negotiation down the side of the table. Now you are ready to evaluate them.

Step 1: Think about the possible outcomes of each alternative. This is best done as a group—discuss together what you think would happen if each alternative was employed.

Step 2: Have each family member rate each alternative with a plus or a minus.

Step 3: For each alternative, score an overall "plus" in the total column if the majority of the group gives it a "plus." Give the alternative a "minus" if the majority of the group does not like the alternative. Using communication skills, discuss and negotiate alternatives with tied scores.

recommend you go through Exercise 9C. A blank worksheet that looks like Table 9.3 that the Changs completed is provided at the end of this book to assist you in listing your family's alternatives.

Did any of your scores on Exercise 9C surprise you? Did you change your mind about any alternatives? Talk this exercise over with your family, and discuss your different reactions.

STEP 4: DECIDING ON A COURSE OF ACTION

Up to this point, you and your family have concentrated on narrowing down a long list of alternatives to only the most promising ones that: 1) involve cooperation and negotiation, 2) meet the approval of a majority of family members, and 3) fulfill criteria deemed important in regard to your family's special priorities. The next step, then, is to choose the best plan to put into action.

In evaluating positive alternatives by specific criteria, a great deal of information is obtained and organized. This information can be useful in helping clarify the best alternative for a given problem. In the case of the Changs, it became clearer from their criteria worksheet that two alternatives were superior to the others: 1) implementing a structured program of productive activities with Mark and 2) hiring a part-time helper to participate with Mark in these activities.

Before examining the merits of these two alternatives, let us first look at those alternatives that fell short of meeting the Changs'

Table 9.3. Using criteria to evaluate alternatives

Criteria	1) Sharon helps	2) Mr. Chang brings work home	3) Grandparents help	4) Part-time constructive helper	5) Continue treatment	6) Consider hospital in 1 month	7) Structured Program
				Alternatives			
Provides long-term progress				X			X
Increases family members' independence				X			X
Will alleviate stress quickly	X	X	X	X	X	X	X
Promotes health and security					X		X
Furthers intellectual/personal growth				X			X
Increases social contact and rewards	X	X	X	X			X
Solves other problems as well				X		X	X
Does not relate to other problems			X	X	X		X
Easy to carry out	X		X		X	X	
Will be enjoyable			X	X			X
Economical	X	X	X				X
Number of criteria met	4	3	6	8	3	2	10

needs. Enlisting the help of Sharon, Mr. Chang, or the Changs' grand-parents clearly had several benefits. These alternatives offered rapid relief to the current stress on Mrs. Chang, expanded Mark's social world, and were easy and economical options. However, they failed to meet two of the Changs' top priorities. They failed both to offer the promise of long-term improvement in Mark's condition and, in fact, *restricted* the independence of Sharon and Mr. Chang. Furthermore, these alternatives were not expected to increase family members'

Exercise 9C

Worksheet 9C is a blank worksheet arranged similarly to the one used by the Chang family in completing this exercise.

Step One: As a family, think of all the possible results of a *perfect* solution to the problem you are addressing. To provide clues, refer to your family values (Chapter 2) and the needs you consider most important (Chapter 5). Put these criteria in the space provided on the worksheet.

Step Two: Look back at your answers in Exercise 9B, and list all the alternatives receiving an overall "plus" rating across the top of the page.

Step Three: Consider which criteria each alternative meets. Place an "X" in the box where the alternative meets the criterion.

Step Four: Put the total number of criteria met by each alternative at the bottom of the page.

---

health, sense of security, or intellectual or personal growth. Thus, this "babysitting" approach to improving the Changs' situation in a satisfactory manner failed to fulfill a number of important criteria.

Similarly, the options of merely continuing current treatment efforts and reconsidering hospitalization in one month met few of the Changs' criteria. Primarily, they failed to alter significantly the current stressful situation and thus failed to provide any immediate or long-term benefits. Although neither of these alternatives could be employed as a primary plan of action, they could be adopted as adjuncts to the final plan. That is, continuing treatment efforts and reconsidering hospitalization are options that are easy to carry out and will not disrupt the more immediate and renewed approach needed to alleviate the current situation.

The Changs' best alternatives consisted of designing a structured program of constructive activities and hiring part-time help. The implementation of a productive program was expected to yield a variety of benefits by: 1) keeping Mark active and alert, 2) allowing less opportunity for destructive thoughts or actions, 3) increasing Mark's sense of competence, worth, and esteem, 4) preparing Mark for eventual employment, and 5) affording Mark and his family the opportunity to develop greater independence and a more satisfying quality of life. In short, this alternative met the Changs' most important criteria promising long-term gains and greater family independence.

Exercise 9D

Using the criteria worksheet completed in Exercise 9C, compare the criteria (and criteria totals) met by each alternative. Does one stand out as superior to the others? If so, are family members in agreement that this is the best alternative? If no one alternative is clearly the best one, discuss which alternative seems to meet the most important criteria. Employ negotiation and communication skills to exchange ideas, work through differences, and arrive at a decision that is acceptable to the majority of those family members involved in the problem-solving process. The end result should be a chosen plan of attack in resolving a current family problem.

In addition, the employment of a part-time helper to spend productive time with Mark fulfilled many of these same criteria. In fact, by combining both alternatives, an even greater number of criteria could be met. Thus, the Changs determined that their best course of action was to hire a competent individual to work with them in developing and implementing a program of structured, growth-oriented activities. Exercise 9D is designed to take your family through the decision-making process used by the Chang family.

In many cases, choosing a plan of action involves a good deal of discussion, negotiation, and open communication among family members. Every family needs to deal with differences of opinion among its members. A step-by-step approach is one way to deal with these differences, because everyone can readily understand the reasons for choosing one course of action over another. You will be surprised at how easily common agreement can be reached. Each individual's perspectives, needs, and values play a crucial role in the ultimate effectiveness of a family solution. Similarly, a systematic and organized approach to problem solving is often the best way to address the many needs that confront families.

CHAPTER

10

Taking Action

Once an alternative or set of alternatives is chosen as the solution for a given problem, your family is ready to take action. This stage, where problems are resolved and needs are met, is often the most exciting and satisfying part of the problem-solving process. Taking action involves three closely related and often overlapping processes that can be undertaken in a series of steps. The first step is to map out a strategy for implementing the solution. Assume, for example, that Mr. and Mrs. Singer (whom we discussed in Chapter 9) decided to seek marital counseling in order to resolve their difficulties. The process of mapping out a step-by-step strategy for implementing this solution requires that the couple determine where to go for counseling, when to arrange sessions, how to handle payment, and so forth. Thus, planning a strategy right down to the step-by-step details is the first task involved in taking action.

Step 2 requires that your family determine who will implement each of the tasks specified in the step-by-step plan. This step is often best accomplished by delegating various responsibilities to individual family members. Thus, in the case of the Singers, Mr. Singer can take responsibility for locating a good marital counselor in town, Mrs. Singer can contact him or her and set up the appointment, and Mr.

Singer can determine if their health insurance covers the counselor's fee. By dividing and sharing the responsibilities involved with implementing a solution, the family ensures an efficient and cooperative effort.

The third step allows family members to carry out their assigned tasks. Springing into action at this point, however, does not put an end to family communication. In fact, it is especially crucial during this phase that members check in with one another on an *ongoing* basis. This type of consistent feedback ensures that "bugs" in the operation receive immediate attention, that new strategies are developed when different needs arise, and that progress is reported and continued as the solution takes effect. Although every solution requires a different degree of step-by-step planning, allocation of responsibilities, and ongoing communication during implementation, these steps are necessary in order to best resolve a problem. Each of these three steps is discussed in greater detail in this chapter, and both exercises and examples are provided to assist your own family in taking action.

Making a decision is not the final step in problem solving. Although agreeing on a final decision may, indeed, be much of the battle, further planning is necessary to determine how a given solution can best be implemented. Consider the following case study.

Mrs. Gonzales is the grandmother of two children under her care. Her grandson Victor is a senior in high school. Her granddaughter Gabriela is 15 years old and moderately retarded. She attends a special class at the high school and is dropped off at home each day at 3 o'clock by a school van. This arrangement has allowed Mrs. Gonzales to work full-time as a bank teller and return home by 4:30 P.M. to attend to her grandchildren.

Recently, Mrs. Gonzales was shocked to hear from Victor that a neighborhood boy had seduced Gabriela in their home that afternoon. Mrs. Gonzales's initial reaction was that of fear, rage, and deep sorrow. After she had calmed herself, she was able to learn from Gabriela and the boy's parents that Gabriela was a willing participant, not a victim of rape. Yet, given the vulnerability of her granddaughter, she was outraged and sought out the support of several close friends and her sister Tina. Once she felt more in control of her emotions and having expressed her anger and sadness, Mrs. Gonzales realized that something needed to be done. She took careful inventory of the situation and discovered that she and her family had many important problems that demanded immediate attention.

Mrs. Gonzales was clearly deeply distressed, not only by this incident but also by her sudden awareness of her granddaughter's sexuality. Despite Gabriela's mental retardation, her granddaughter was becoming a woman physically and emotionally. Mrs. Gonzales was embarrassed to realize that she had never thought it necessary to educate Gabriela about sex, just as her own mother had neglected to educate her. Nonetheless, this oversight had done little to thwart Gabriela's sexual feelings or reproductive capabilities.

After talking about the incident with Victor and Gabriela, Mrs. Gonzales identified three needs to address immediately: 1) Gabriela needed to be educated, not only about the physiological aspects of sex but about emotional and social aspects as well; 2) Gabriela needed some form of birth control; and 3) Gabriela needed more supervision around men. The question still remained, however, how the Gonzales's could accomplish these three goals.

First, Mrs. Gonzales sought information from her priest, a close friend, and her family physician. After brainstorming and evaluating numerous alternatives with the help of these resource persons and her grandchildren, the Gonzales family decided on three alternatives to meet the three needs. First, it was decided that she herself would talk with Gabriela about sex. Second, a decision was made that although sterilization was a potential alternative in the future, for now Gabriela would begin taking birth control pills as a precaution. Third, Victor would take responsibility for staying with his sister from 3:00 to 4:30 P.M. 3 afternoons a week, and Tina would take over the other 2 days so Victor could attend wrestling practice. Thus, the Gonzales's had made several decisions concerning the issue of Gabriela's sexual vulnerability. Much of the work, however, had only just begun.

Although the chosen alternatives were clearly identified, a number of associated questions regarding their actual implementation remained unanswered. For example, where and when was Mrs. Gonzales to obtain sex information materials? Exactly what message did she want to communicate to Gabriela? When and where should Gabriela be taken to have birth control pills prescribed? What rules regarding afternoon visitors did she want to work out with Gabriela and Victor? Thus, it was still necessary for the Gonzales's to examine each of the chosen solutions and break them down further into step-by-step plans of action.

The case of the Gonzales family helps to illustrate the importance of developing a step-by-step plan when taking action in a problematic situation. How can a family accomplish this?

STEP 1: DEVELOPING A STEP-BY-STEP PLAN OF ACTION

It is helpful to consider the input of as many family members as possible when choosing a strategy for implementing a solution. In addition, members of your larger social support network can be particularly helpful at this point. Contacting that friend whose own daughter is seeing a therapist in order to obtain a referral or that neighbor who is handy around her house for hints about installing a ramp can provide key information about how best to implement a solution. Determining a strategy for action relies on the input and suggestions of family members. Thus, brainstorming skills are often used at this step in the problem-solving process as well.

First, family members need to identify those aspects of the solution that need further specification and planning. For example, if a solution calls for purchasing a motorized wheelchair, factors still requiring planning may include: 1) who will pick it out, 2) what type to purchase, 3) how much to spend, 4) how to pay for it, and 5) when to buy it. Once these aspects of a solution are identified, the family can reemploy the problem-solving process in order to meet these mini-needs. Thus, families need to identify and resolve those issues upon which solutions hinge.

Once your family has developed a plan for carrying out each phase of the solution, it is helpful to conceptualize the overall plan into a series of steps. Thus, for building a wheelchair-accessible ramp, a family's list of steps may look something like this:

1. Determine the best location to install the ramp.
2. Check out library books on home carpentry.
3. Ask Mr. and Mrs. O'Connor for details on their ramp.
4. Purchase wood at lumberyard.
5. Call Frank and set up a time he can help.
6. Get a babysitter for the kids on Saturday and Sunday morning.

Breaking a plan down into its components makes its implementation easier and ensures a better outcome in the long run. Exercise 10A is designed to help your family with such step-by-step planning.

Quite possibly, while completing Exercise 10A, you discovered that family members do not always have identical points of view. It is heartening, however, to find that it is possible to reach a compromise in most situations and still meet the larger goal of solving the issue at

Exercise 10A

Using the solution your family chose to resolve a family problem in Exercise 9D, complete the following steps:

Step 1: Discuss and specify steps of the solution that need further planning.

Step 2: Brainstorm alternative plans for implementing each step of the plan.

Step 3: Evaluate each alternative by discussion and/or ratings. Negotiate a mutually agreeable plan for each phase of the solution.

hand. The case of the Gonzales family further illustrates the importance of step-by-step planning during the process of taking action.

Although Mrs. Gonzales had decided that some form of sex education was necessary for her granddaughter, she was uncertain how exactly she should proceed. First, she asked Gabriela if she would like to talk to the doctor about the incident with the boy. Gabriela stated that she wanted to talk with her grandmother only. Mrs. Gonzales then recontacted the physician and asked what she should tell a young woman with an intellectual disability. The physician frankly admitted that he was uncertain about what information Gabriela could best use and suggested that Mrs. Gonzales speak with Gabriela's schoolteacher. In addition, he gave her the names and phone numbers of two families for first-hand advice about raising mentally retarded adolescents. At that point, Mrs. Gonzales felt ready to break down her sex education plan into a step-by-step process. She wrote down the following list of tasks:

1. *Set aside next Saturday morning.*
2. *Go to public library and look through available books.*
3. *Schedule an appointment with Gabriela's teacher.*
4. *Contact the recommended families by phone.*
5. *Jot down the most basic and essential information in simple language that Gabriela can understand.*
6. *Select a mutually agreeable time with Gabriela to talk.*
7. *Talk with Gabriela and explore her feelings concerning the incident, her sexuality, and marriage.*

*Thus, Mrs. Gonzales worked out a detailed plan by which to imple-
ment one phase of the plan of action.*

Often, it is not feasible for one family member to assume
responsibility for both designing and implementing a plan of action. In
such cases, it is valuable to enlist as many family members as possible
and to draw on members in your social and formal support networks as
well. Each individual can be useful in suggesting steps in the solution,
and discussion can determine the best step-by-step procedures. Then,
each member can be assigned responsibility for one or more steps.

STEP 2:   ASSIGNING AND ASSUMING RESPONSIBILITY

Within families, a constant process of give-and-take occurs as members help to meet each others' daily and long-range needs. It is this
curious combination of independence and interdependence that is so
essential to our well-being. We learn to rely on each other and to
reciprocate in our own special ways. In order to complete a family
task, family members need to combine their varied resources of
energy, time, know-how, encouragement, and material support. Thus,
once a step-by-step plan is designed, implementing it involves enlisting the participation of family members.

How can responsibilities be delegated fairly? This question can
only be answered on an individual basis, for what is a fair amount of
responsibility to one person may seem burdensome to another. Family
members need to take stock of their individual strengths and resources and then capitalize upon them by assuming appropriate responsibilities. Thus, the voluntary contribution of each member's
talents is perhaps the ideal way to allocate responsibilities.

Exercise 10B can help your family implement the step-by-step
plan you created in Exercise 10A. Answering the questions in the
exercise should help your family distribute responsibilities fairly and
wisely.

Individual strengths are just one consideration in assuming
responsibility. Often, taking responsibility involves merely filling in
where one is needed, even on an unsavory chore. The willingness,
then, to give of oneself in a group effort is central to the successful
resolution of family needs. Few families, however, always live up to
this high ideal of unselfish cooperation. More often than not, family
members need to negotiate their portion of responsibility until a fair
arrangement has been made. Because of family members' differences
of opinion and need, often the fullest cooperation arises from sincere

Exercise 10B

Using your step-by-step plan mapped out in Exercise 10A, assemble the family and assign responsibility for steps within the plan to individual family members. During the entire procedure, pay careful attention to communication patterns within the family. As individuals, ask the following questions: How are conflicts handled? Does one person dominate discussion or remain conspicuously quiet? Are differences of opinion negotiated to a satisfactory compromise? Is each person satisfied with the task assignments? Discuss your individual answers to these questions as a family.

and deliberate efforts at communication. The following case study exemplifies the cooperation of a family striving to meet its needs through interdependence and the careful allocation of individual resources.

Sam Fontaine, age 42, was recently disabled when a drunken driver collided with his car. In that accident, Mr. Fontaine suffered spinal cord damage and is now paralyzed below the waist. His wife Marilyn and their two sons Joe, age 21, and Frank, 17, have all pitched in to fulfill some of Mr. Fontaine's previous responsibilities. Mrs. Fontaine took on a part-time waitressing job, while Joe, a mechanic, has contributed to the family income. Frank took over much of the maintenance around the house.

Since the accident, Mr. Fontaine has grown increasingly depressed and despondent. Having lost his sense of independence and accompanying feelings of competence and worth, Mr. Fontaine considers himself a burden on the family and misses both his role as breadwinner and his vocation as a locksmith. During a recent family rap session, Mr. Fontaine expressed his distress at losing these roles within the family. He asked his family for suggestions to help him develop a plan for becoming both active and financially productive again. After extensive information gathering, discussion, brainstorming, and evaluation of alternatives, the Fontaines decided to undertake a small family locksmith business.

As you might expect, in order to undertake such an extensive project, the Fontaines needed to develop a detailed step-by-step procedure and to delegate a number of important responsibilities before their plan could actually be implemented. Thus, the Fontaines all worked together in planning and in assuming responsibilities within the plan. For example, Mr. Fontaine, who has extensive knowledge and contact with other locksmiths, assumed responsibility for all business planning, as well as for getting advice from his former boss and colleagues. Joe, the oldest and most mechanically minded of the two boys, was placed in charge of stock and home repairs. Frank was made both Joe's and Mr. Fontaine's assistant, because he felt he would prefer less responsibility in light of his other activities. Mrs. Fontaine, who managed the household finances, was placed in charge of the bookkeeping.

The family business plan thus required that the Fontaines all work together. It also served the added purpose of increasing each member's independence, whether emotionally (i.e., Mr. Fontaine), financially (i.e., Joe and Frank), or in terms of choosing a more familiar and convenient lifestyle (i.e., Mrs. Fontaine). Thus, the process of independence often evolves out of a spirit of interdependence, where family resources are combined and ultimately enhanced.

STEP 3:   GO TO WORK, BUT STAY IN TOUCH!

Wouldn't it be wonderful if our problems always managed to disappear with good planning and effort? Although they often do, at times new problems emerge without warning. Similarly, a chosen solution may sometimes need to be reassessed if it is not working to our satisfaction. For example, in the case of the Fontaines, it can be expected that, despite their preliminary plans and efforts, the complexity of starting a family business is apt to pose new challenges periodically. Thus, it is imperative to view problem solving as an *ongoing* process. Problem-solving skills, once learned, can consistently be applied toward meeting the many needs of a family over time.

Once a plan of action has been put into effect, it is important that family members continue to communicate on a regular basis. Such ongoing discussion can help pinpoint areas of progress or sources of delay in carrying through a plan of action. Thus, communication can help "nip in the bud" those aspects of a plan that are not working. For example, assume that in the Fontaine family Frank decides that his responsibility as an employee is interfering with his social activities. By voicing this dissatisfaction, the family can identify a new problem and begin brainstorming alternatives to meet both the needs of Frank and the family business *before* the problem worsens.

An even more important reason to provide ongoing feedback is to allow family members to share the fantastic feelings of success that come with meeting needs and solving problems. As the long-awaited ramp is being built, the family member is becoming educated, or the overworked individual is gaining relief, the enthusiastic communication of progress and success provides a boost for everyone. Such verbal sharing can prevent discouragement among members and actually can increase the rate of progress toward a problem's end.

Although it may be discouraging to realize that some first-strike attacks against particularly stubborn problems may not always bring success, it is encouraging to know that it is not necessary to carry out a chosen plan to the bitter end. That is, it is always possible to try a new alternative solution, fine-tune the current one, or pick up the problem-solving process at an earlier phase. As an ongoing process, problem solving does not always flow smoothly to easy success without some coaxing and attention. Successful problem solving often takes hard work and cooperation. Fortunately, the benefit of utilizing a problem-solving approach is often seen in the direct and rapid resolution of many family problems.

In summary, there are three steps involved in taking effective action. First, mapping out a step-by-step strategy helps ensure that the solution is carefully and smoothly implemented. Second, distributing responsibilities for these tasks among family members helps capitalize on family strengths while maximizing efficiency. Third, actually carrying out the plan constitutes the "coup de grace" of family problem solving. This final stage, when problems are resolved, relies heavily on the communication and support your family provides its members. After this point, your family is ready to tackle new problems or simply enjoy the added freedom and independence that problem resolution brings.

CHAPTER

11

Taking Charge
Meeting Needs, Solving Problems

You and your family have special needs that may stem from illness or disability in a family member. Often, these special needs may feel intolerable, overwhelming, and unresolvable. Disability and chronic illness can appear to be all-encompassing circumstances that complicate and blacken all aspects of your life. And sometimes a disability or illness can be experienced as a tragedy that leaves your family without hope, power, or resource. These feelings are very real and deeply valid. Yet the question remains: What can we do about these feelings and circumstances? This book asserts a single answer: Plenty.

Each of the six families introduced at the beginning of the book, as well as the many other families we have come to know, experienced their own unique struggles in coming to grips with the onset of illness or disability in a family member. Their examples teach us many things. Indeed, life is unpredictable, and we cannot hope to control all its twists and turns. Yet, although we cannot design and choreograph all the circumstances of our lives, we do have the crucial power to determine how we respond to and cope with the challenges we face. The manner in which we identify and respond to the special needs generated by an illness or disability (e.g., mobility, special education, finances, despair, medical care, or stress) empowers us with the ability to substantially lessen the negative impact of unforeseen events.

This book has engaged you in a challenge. Not only have you taken stock of your family's untapped resources but you have also embarked on a process of taking charge of your life. This process, called problem solving, requires that you harness your many resources and launch a concerted effort aimed at meeting family needs and resolving family problems. The prerequisite for success in such a powerful endeavor stems from understanding that your family is its own best decision maker and your willingness to take responsibility and control. These problem-solving attitudes are deceptively straight-forward. Each of us grapples daily with asserting our needs and assuming responsibility for ensuring that they are met, and this is no easy task. Learning that you are in charge is a slow and painful process, and indeed, many individuals never attain this insight. By virtue of your interest in this book and in solving the problems in your family's life, we are well aware of your willingness to face the obstacles and problems you confront. This, we assert, is more than half the battle. And the steps we have guided you through in the problem-solving process is your victory lap.

You began this book by examining the many strengths and resources available to you and your family. Some of these were easy to identify: tangible skills, financial resources, or smarts, to name but a few. Others, however, required some searching on your part until you were able to draw into your wellspring the many assets you have taken for granted or overlooked. Courage, stamina, creativity, under-standing, spiritual strengths, time, patience, hope, willpower, or special talents may be the strengths you have just begun to acknowl-edge and thus add to your arsenal of coping devices. You may have discovered strength and guidance merely by listing and thinking about your personal values. Or you may have gained insight into the pri-orities of other family members whose values differ from your own. Taking stock of your values and resources is the starting point for coping with and meeting needs.

We have also asked you to look beyond your own family to take stock of the resources in your community. Social and formal support systems can complement and fortify your family's own reserves by providing material, emotional, or informational support. Friends, neighbors and relatives can all play an important role in helping you solve, as well as avoid problems. Clearly, developing an active social life or a strong reciprocal relationship of give-and-take is complicated by many factors. Some families are terribly busy, and time may not allow for extensive socializing. Other families are uncomfortable with the stigma they perceive and may withdraw from relationships as a result. And still other families value their privacy and prefer to keep to themselves. None of these conflicts need interfere with building and maintaining the kind of social support your family deserves. In fact, by following three suggestions, you may be better able to create important ties that you have never thought possible. Providing information about disability or chronic illness to relatives and friends can lessen fears, facilitate awareness, and thus overcome stigma. Practicing reciprocity can strengthen your social system, as well as ensure the maximal use of your time and resources. Perhaps most important, emphasizing the strengths of the chronically ill or disabled member can help others see beyond stereotypes and stigma into the most genuine and positive aspects of your family.

Often, we reach beyond both our families and our social support networks for the varied resources that professionals can provide. Physicians, psychologists, teachers, social workers, and the like all exist to meet families' needs. If you are experienced in working with professionals, you are well aware that it often takes assertiveness, courtesy, and perseverance to secure the help you need. Professionals are human, and they often amaze or disappoint us as such. By seeking out competent help, you may find formal support to be an invaluable resource for meeting family needs.

How can having a family member with an illness or disability affect family needs? There is no universal answer to this question, and we have therefore asked that you examine the needs of your own family. Perhaps you have a chronic illness and find that some needs have increased and others have become less intense. Or you may have a loved one with a disability and find that some of your needs conflict with theirs. Your experience with family needs reflects that: 1) all families have a variety of needs and emphasize each to greater or lesser degrees, 2) all members' needs are important, and 3) each family member's needs affect those of other members as well. Understanding the individuality and relatedness of family needs is extremely helpful to the communication and problem solving that must take place if needs are to be met fairly. All families work hard at meeting needs on a daily basis. Sometimes, however, the normal course of family activities does not address certain important needs. These unmet needs can often fester and magnify if they are not identified and actively addressed. They can thus rapidly become problems.

Herein lies the focus of this book: family problem solving. Problem solving is the active, ongoing process by which individuals, groups, and families identify a problem and systematically work out a solution. Whether a problem involves housing, medical care, dwindling self-esteem, lost hope, financial worries, transportation, or family conflict, problem solving can often be used to a satisfying end. Throughout the problem-solving process, good communication has served as the password to success. Good communication is not an ideal reserved for talented public speakers or group therapy participants. Rather, it always involves an individual style that combines heart and mind messages that fit with the personality of the communicator. Such varied styles of good communication do, however, contain common elements. Effective communication involves the use of constructive statements that express your needs and feelings in a clear, direct, and nonthreatening manner. Similarly, on the flip side of communication, active listening requires attention, clarification, and acceptance of others' perspectives. By examining your own family's communication patterns you have taken a difficult step that can yield lifelong pay-offs. Working toward good communication is not an easy process, but just as all families have strengths, they all have the potential to express themselves in an effective and rewarding manner.

Good communication can greatly facilitate the identification of troublesome issues or problems in your family. Each member has both the right and responsibility to express his or her needs and identify situations that require change. Once a problem is thus aired, problem solving can progress to the stage of generating ideas and alternatives that might be a solution. This process, called brainstorming, only requires an open mind and the active involvement of as many family members and resource persons as possible. The goal of brainstorming is not to produce the best solution, but to generate a quantity of spontaneous ideas. In fact, at this stage, it is important that family members do not evaluate their ideas in any way. The goal is to encourage creativity and the free-flowing expression of ideas.

Once your family has generated a list of alternatives, you can begin to evaluate them systematically. This step leads to the selection of one best alternative that is ultimately implemented. In choosing an alternative, your family draws again from values and priorities to evaluate the desirability of outcomes that may result from various plans of action. By using communication skills, open discussion, and negotiation, families can determine the best recourse against a particular problem.

Taking action is often the most exciting stage in the problem-solving process. As needs are met and problems resolved, the deep satisfaction of positive change adds to your family's feelings of success. Taking action requires that family members keep in close touch as they devise a step-by-step plan of action; establish a division of labor and resources; and pursue ongoing communication, evaluation, and feedback. Thus, problem solving is an ongoing, fluid process. It does not stop once action has begun or even once change is first noted. Rather, you should return to each of the problem-solving steps as new situations and new alternatives come into play.

Problem solving is a skill that improves dramatically with practice. In time, you and your family may find yourselves using various aspects of the problem-solving process automatically and instinctively. What we have hoped to provide here is a guide to the structure and process of problem solving. Undoubtedly, your family will adapt this process to your own unique style of tackling problems and meeting needs.

In rising to the many challenges we have put forth in this book, you have gained more than simply a tool for solving problems. You have, in fact, taken charge of your life. It is our hope that you will take heart in the powers you possess. The power to choose, the strength to control how you respond to and face challenge, is the power to change your world. We have not sought to minimize the concerns you hold nor the troubles that you face. Rather, we have encouraged you to fully grasp and maximize the strengths and assets you possess. For those of you seeking to wholeheartedly love, care for, and live with family members with special needs, we invite you to take stock of your many resources and harness your varied potentials. In this way, you can conquer circumstances, defeat despair, and thrive despite adversity.

APPENDIX

Resources

CRITERIA FOR INCLUSION

Listed below are recommended readings that you may find helpful. Several important criteria were used to select the items listed under each topic area. First, the material is written in a clear, readable, and accessible style. Second, it addresses a broad variety of disabilities and chronic illnesses, as well as different age groups. Third, the chosen resources are readily available, either through the ordering information provided, the publisher, a library, or bookstore. Also included in the final section is a brief list of organizations that you may be interested in contacting for further information, as well as several books that provide more extensive listings than the ones we have included here. The recommended readings are divided into 10 areas:

- A. Personal accounts
- B. Financial planning and guardianship
- C. Daily physical needs
- D. Recreational needs
- E. Affectional needs and sexuality
- F. Education
- G. Communication

H. Stress and coping
I. Comprehensive resource guides
J. Organizations

A. PERSONAL ACCOUNTS

These books draw on the deep insight and valuable knowledge of individuals' own experiences with disability and chronic illness. Each of these selections provides honest, moving, and often inspiring personal accounts of life with special needs.

1. Turnbull, H. R., & Turnbull, A. P. (Eds.). (1985). *Parents speak out: Then and now* (2nd ed.). Columbus, OH: Charles E. Merrill. $11.95.

    This is a unique book that includes original essays by authors who are both professionals in the disability field and parents of disabled children. A powerful message is conveyed that the entire family needs help with feelings and must learn to acknowledge anger, as well as to communicate joy and the sense of challenge. Other issues explored include the relationship between parent and professional, the transition of the disabled child into adulthood, the stresses associated with institutionalization and deinstitutionalization, and the importance of other family members' needs. The authors' contributions are honest and emotionally rich. These are essays about years of hard battle and moments of exquisite joy.

2. Zola, I. K. (1982). *Missing pieces*. Philadelphia: Temple University Press. $9.95.

    Missing Pieces is a personal chronicle of life with a disability. Irving Zola describes four processes toward independence he discovered as a physically disabled individual. These involve overcoming the denial of one's sexuality, anger, vulnerability, and potentiality. A truly sensitive, inspiring, and moving autobiographical account.

3. Harris, G. A. (1983). *Broken ears, wounded hearts*. Washington, DC: Gallaudet College Press. $10.95.

    Written by the father of a hearing-impaired daughter, *Broken Ears* portrays the persistent search of a young couple to discover what is wrong with their child and then to cope with "wounded hearts." This book also portrays how a father grew as much as his daughter, although not without pain and sacrifice. Through both agonizing and joyful times, George Harris's perseverance and depth of caring provide hope to all present and prospective parents.

4. Orlansky, M. D., & Heward, W. L. (1981). *Voices: Interviews with handicapped people.* Columbus, OH: Charles E. Merrill. $10.95.

    This book provides a forum for children and adults with disabilities to express their own points of view based on their own experiences. A wide variety of individuals of different ages, educational backgrounds, economic status, ethnic origins, and types and severity of disability are interviewed. The result is a series of conversations with diverse individuals who both enrich our knowledge and touch us deeply. As stated by the authors, the goal of *Voices* is for readers to "come to know a disabled individual as a person, not just as a 'case of disability.' "

5. Featherstone, H. (1982). *A difference in the family: Living with a disabled child.* New York: Penguin Books. $4.95.

    This is a highly compassionate account that traces the long road toward acceptance of a disability. The author, an educator and mother of a severely disabled child, discusses how parents and siblings can cope with their feelings of fear, anger, guilt, and loneliness. She also explains what types of support and understanding can be provided by professionals. Many people whose lives have been touched by a physically or mentally disabled child will find reassurance and invaluable guidance in this book.

6. Kushner, H. S. (1981). *When bad things happen to good people.* New York: Avon. $3.50.

    This book is a biographical account of a clergyman's son who died from a rare disease. The author describes the impact his son's death had on his feelings about God and his own religion. He also describes the process he went through to come to terms with his family's tragedy. This is a very moving and sensitive piece of work.

7. Deford, F. (1983). *Alex: The life of a child.* New York: Viking Press. $13.95.

    This moving book is the story of Alex, a young girl with cystic fibrosis, who had a special gift for human insight. Written by Alex's dad, this book provides a rare view into the life of a family who faced chronic illness and death. The impact of Alex's illness and death on her mother, father, and brother is poignantly described, along with the family's interactions with doctors and involvement in medical intervention. Frank Deford's feelings about his daughter and his own grief and faith are generously shared, along with Alex's courage and love.

B. FINANCIAL PLANNING AND GUARDIANSHIP

The selected resources in this section provide information on estate planning, guardianship, money management, and insurance issues relevant to families with disabled members.

1. Fruge, D. L., & Green, K. O. (1982). *Estate planning for retarded persons and their families.* Atlanta: University of Mississippi Law Center. $7.95.

    This book provides information for parents and guardians on the legal issues involved in estate planning for retarded citizens and their families. Much of the information, however, is also applicable to persons with other disabilities or illnesses that limit their ability to care for themselves. Chapters cover issues pertaining to government assistance, guardianships, estate planning, wills, trusts, life insurance, annuities, and more.

2. Russell, L. M. (1983). *Alternatives: A family guide to legal and financial planning for the disabled.* Evanston, IL: First Publications. $11.95.

    Alternatives includes chapters on the varied elements of planning for individuals with mental disabilities: wills, guardianship, trusts, government benefits, taxes, insurance, and financial planning. The special needs of families with mentally disabled members are discussed clearly and frankly, and numerous angles to estate planning are explored. Importantly, this book helps families plan early and carefully, making the personal and financial planning processes understandable and adaptable to the individual needs of families.

3. United Cerebral Palsy of Minnesota, Inc. (1983). *Health care coverage and your disabled child.* St. Paul, MN: Author.

    This simple pamphlet covers basic, yet important, issues related to obtaining and using health care coverage. A question-and-answer format is used during the first half of the pamphlet (e.g., How do I file a claim? Will my insurance coverage pay for my child's electric wheelchair?). Then, a discussion of various health care options, including private health insurance, health maintenance organizations, and public plans, is provided. Contact: United Cerebral Palsy of Minnesota, 1821 Univ. Ave., Rm. 233 South, St. Paul, MN 55104 (612) 646-7588.

C. DAILY PHYSICAL NEEDS

The following selections focus on time management, a skill all of us employ to varying degrees of success as we carry out our daily activities. Guidelines for caring for the physical needs of individuals with certain disabilities are also covered.

1. Fraser, B. A., & Hensinger, R. N. (1983). *Managing physical handicaps: A practical guide for parents, care providers, and educators.* Baltimore: Paul H. Brookes Publishing Co. $19.95.

    This is a complete and well-illustrated practical reference, resource, and guide for the care and management of individuals with disabilities. This book ultilizes a problem-solving approach to help parents, educators, and caretakers in the day-to-day care of individuals with severe physical disabilities. The authors translate confusing terminology into easy-to-understand language and offer a myriad of practical suggestions. A glossary is included, as well as more than 100 illustrations.

2. Lakein, A. (1973). *How to get control of your time and your life.* New York: Signet. $2.50.

    This book is a practical guide to managing your personal and business time. In short, concise chapters, Lakein discusses how to set short-term and long-term goals, establish priorities, organize a daily schedule, and achieve better self-understanding. Guidelines are also suggested to help build willpower, create quiet time, and approach unpleasant tasks. This is a handy guide that can help individuals and families better accomplish their goals.

3. Winston, S. (1978). *Getting organized: The easy way to put your life in order.* New York: W. W. Norton. $12.95.

    This is a very helpful, practical guide to organizing time amidst the demands of home and work. Sections are devoted to time, paperwork, money, and the home.

4. Finnie, N. R. (1975). *Handling the young cerebral palsied child at home.* New York: Dutton. $6.50.

This is a very practical guide for parents, nurses, doctors, therapists, social workers and others involved in caring for young children with cerebral palsy. Chapters cover the broad physical needs of the child, from principles of handling and movement to feeding, toilet training, and bathing. A guide to community resources and suppliers of accessories and equipment is also included.

5. Power, P. W., & Dell Orto, A. E. (1980). *Role of the family in the rehabilitation of the physically disabled.* Baltimore: University Park Press. $23.95.

This comprehensive book explores the family's role in coping with physical disability. A broad range of disabilities are examined in terms of their unique effects on families at different points throughout the life cycle. *Role of the Family* explores the complex family dynamics that affect problems relating to a family member's disability. Numerous case studies and personal vignettes are used to illustrate the social, behavioral, psychological, and medical impacts of physical disability. Intervention strategies, coping mechanisms, and stress mediation techniques are a valuable part of the discussion.

D. RECREATIONAL NEEDS

The need of all individuals to enjoy recreational activities is addressed in each of these selections. Suggestions and resources are provided to help you meet your own recreational needs.

1. Wuerch, B. B., & Voeltz, L. M. (1982). *Longitudinal leisure skills for severely handicapped learners: The Ho'onanea curriculum component.* Baltimore: Paul H. Brookes Publishing Co. $17.95.

Longitudinal Leisure Skills describes a lifelong leisure skills curriculum component for learners with severe disabilities. Focusing on the personal preferences and needs of students and their families, the Ho'onanea program balances the traditional curriculum emphasis on such areas as self-help, language, and gross motor skills with an equivalent concern for constructive use of leisure time to enhance the overall quality of students' lives. The Ho'onanea program is designed to help students decrease inappropriate behaviors, strengthen skills, and enhance successful community adjustment.

2. Schechter, D., Sygall, S., & Powell, K. (1982). Recreation and social activities. In A. H. Katz & K. Martin (Eds.), *A Handbook of services for the handicapped* (pp. 211–236). Westport, CT: Greenwood Press. $35.00.

    This is an extremely useful chapter that discusses the range of recreation and social activities available to persons with disabilities. From nature tours, basketball, bowling, and square dancing to skiing, ping pong, running, and the arts, this material provides an extensive list of suggestions and resources for refreshing one's mind and body through recreation and social activity.

3. Fluegelman, A. (1976). *New games book.* New York: Doubleday. $7.95.

    This book focuses on playing games for fun, emphasizing cooperation, not competition. New games are intended to improve physical health and stamina in a relaxed, enjoyable, and nonstrenuous manner.

E. AFFECTIONAL NEEDS AND SEXUALITY

The important need of all individuals for affection is addressed in the following selections that focus on sexuality and disability or illness. Personal insights, legal information, and educational suggestions are provided.

1. Bullard, D., & Knight, S. E. (1981). *Sexuality and physical disability: Personal perspectives.* St. Louis, MO: C. Mosby. $19.95.

    Sexuality and both physical disability and illness are discussed in this book from personal perspectives of individuals, parents, children, and professionals. Contributors, the majority of whom are disabled, offer knowledgeable and poignant insights into being sexual and disabled. A wide range of disabilities is represented, including spinal cord injury, cerebral palsy, ostomy, visual impairment, and mastectomy.

2. Haavik, S. F., & Menninger, K. A. (1981). *Sexuality, law, and the developmentally disabled person: Legal and clinical aspects of marriage, parenthood, and sterilization.* Baltimore: Paul H. Brookes Publishing Co. $15.95.

    This detailed book addresses the difficult questions concerning sexual expression in developmentally disabled adolescents and adults. These complicated issues are fully explored from both clinical and legal perspectives, providing viable options for individualized ways of dealing with questions of sexuality, marriage, procreation, and sterilization. Written by and primarily for professionals, this book provides legal information to strengthen advocacy efforts on the part of developmentally disabled persons.

3. McKee, L., & Blacklidge, V. (1981). *An easy guide for caring parents: Sexuality and socialization.* Contra Costa, CA: Planned Parenthood of Contra Costa. $4.95.

This book, written for parents of people with intellectual disabilities, discusses how to communicate important issues related to sexuality to adolescents and young adults. Masturbation, appropriate social behavior, contraception, marriage, and problems related to sexual activities are a few of the issues addressed in this concise, easy-to-read guide.

F. EDUCATION

The often-frustrating task of obtaining optimal educational opportunities for a disabled family member is made less confusing by the information provided in the following helpful resources.

1. Winton, P. J., Turnbull, A. P., & Blacher, J. (1984). *Selecting a preschool: A guide for parents of handicapped children.* Austin, TX: Pro-Ed. $14.95.

This sensitive book provides parents with practical information for choosing a preschool for their handicapped son or daughter. Information on mainstreaming, special services, and parent involvement activities is provided to help you make the best match between the needs of your child, yourself, and the preschool programs in your community. Chapters are also included on legal rights, involvement in individualized education program (IEP) conferences, and strategies for monitoring your child's preschool program.

2. Turnbull, H., & Turnbull, A. P. (1982). *Free appropriate public education: Law and implementation.* Denver: Love Publishing Co. $9.95.

This book, written by a lawyer and a special education professor who are parents of a disabled child, discusses equal education opportunities for disabled children and youth. Specific principles and cases of federal legislation that speak most directly to the rights of disabled children are presented in detail, along with the steps parents and schools follow in implementing the child's right to free appropriate education. Resistance to such rights are explored, with the authors freely admitting their own biases.

3. Cutler, B. (1981). *Unraveling the special education maze: An action guide for parents.* Champaign, IL: Research Press. $8.95.

    This is a useful guide for parents and professionals alike, elaborating the steps parents must take to ensure that their children receive the services to which they are entitled. This is a very helpful book for parents of school-age children who are either mentally or physically disabled.

4. Shure, M. B., & Spivack, G. (1978). *Problem-solving techniques in childrearing.* San Francisco: Jossey-Bass. $19.95.

    This book focuses on how parents can affect the behavior of their children by encouraging the development of cognitive problem-solving skills. Research data, examples, and exercises are included.

G. COMMUNICATION

The following selections are helpful guides to improving your communication with family members and professionals.

1. Strayhorn, J. M. (1977). *Talking it out: A guide to effective communication and problem solving.* Champaign, IL: Research Press. $7.95.

    This is a highly readable guide to basic principles and strategies of communication and negotiation. Active listening techniques, facilitative versus obstructive messages, "I" statements, and negotiation skills are a few of the communication elements discussed. Dr. Strayhorn includes exercises and humorous examples designed to help the reader employ these skills in real-life situations.

2. Fisher, R., & Ury, W. (1983). *Getting to yes.* New York: Penguin Books. $4.95.

    Getting to Yes presents a step-by-step strategy for coming to mutually acceptable agreements in conflict situations. Based on the work of the Harvard Negotiation Project, this book emphasizes an objective, no-nonsense approach to negotiation.

3. McKay, M., Davis, M., & Fanning, P. (1983). *Messages: The communication book.* Oakland, CA: New Harbinger Publications. $9.95.

   This is a comprehensive guide to personal communication. Basic, advanced, conflict, social, family, and public communication skills are presented in a highly readable and encouraging manner. Exercises and examples are provided to make this handbook a practical, individualized guide.

4. Bach, G. R., & Wyden, P. (1970). *The intimate enemy: How to fight fair in love and marriage.* New York: Avon. $3.95.

   Written primarily for couples, but useful for anyone involved in an interpersonal relationship, *The Intimate Enemy* focuses on strategies for successful, growth-oriented "fair-fighting." This book discusses anger as a natural emotion, the expression of which can be highly productive when done in a skillful manner.

H.   STRESS AND COPING

These resources are highly recommended as aids to your efforts to cope with stresses of life in a healthy and rewarding fashion.

1. Tubesing, D. A. (1981). *Kicking your stress habits: A do-it-yourself guide for coping with stress.* New York: Signet. $2.95.

   This book represents a simple program for recognizing and countering the harmful effects of stress. Written by a psychologist, this book discusses the many forms stress can take and the many ways we can control stress in our own lives.

2. Pelletier, K. (1977). *Mind as healer, mind as slayer (a holistic approach to preventing stress disorders).* New York: Dell. $9.95.

   This book addresses the association between emotional life stress and physical illness. Cardiovascular disease, cancer, arthritis, and respiratory disease are examined, and both the sources of stress, as well as recommendations for the prevention of these stress-related diseases, are provided. The author applies knowledge of stress to the medical practices of today and outlines holistic methods for preventing stress-related illness. This book emphasizes the positive steps that people can take to prevent illness and increase their enjoyment of life.

3. Davis, M., Eshelvrand, E. R., & McKay, M. (1980). *The relaxation and stress reduction workbook*. Richmond, CA: New Harbinger Publications. $11.50.

   This workbook enables readers to choose from a wide variety of techniques for coping with life stress. Progressive relaxation, self-hypnosis, meditation, autogenics, imagination, nutrition, assertiveness training, biofeedback, time management, and exercise are all described in a simple, step-by-step fashion. A very readable and easy-to-use guide, this book provides something for everybody on his or her way to achieving relaxation in the face of stress.

4. Stroebel, C. F. (1982). *QR: The quieting reflex*. New York: Berkley Books. $2.95.

   The quieting reflex (QR) is introduced in this book as a means of countering the harmful physical and psychological effects of stress. The relationship between emotional stress and physical illness is discussed, and QR is presented in a series of easy-to-follow steps. QR involves an awareness of stress in your body and behavior and the ability to overcome it through relaxation and imagery techniques. The ultimate goal of the training provided in this book is to achieve an automatic, 6-second relaxation response to stress, similar to biofeedback without the equipment.

5. Eisenberg, M. G., Sutkin, L. F., & Jansen, M. A. (Eds.). (1984). *Chronic illness and disability through the life span: Effects on self and family* (Vol. 4). New York: Springer Publishing. $23.95.

   Issues that families face as they pass through each life stage are addressed in this book. Reviews of available research are also included. The authors' information is based on their actual clinical experiences. In addition, they examine factors that have contributed to successful coping with chronic illness and disability.

6. Travis, G. (1976). *Chronic illness in children: Its impact on child and family*. Stanford, CA: Stanford University Press. $27.95.

   This book provides information on the psychosocial and medical realities that face families with a chronically ill member. The effects of a family member with a chronic illness on the family as a whole are described from the point of diagnosis throughout the life span. Recommendations are provided to help families cope with their feelings.

7. Moos, R. H. (1977). *Coping with physical illness*. New York: Plenum Medical Book Co. $20.95.

This book includes contributions from a variety of medical and mental health professionals who provide insight into how people cope with serious physical illness. *Coping with Physical Illness* offers a positive emphasis on the human ability to cope with life crises, including a variety of illnesses, such as cancer, severe burns, heart attacks, strokes, and chronic conditions in children. The value of support from family, friends, and community resources is also explored. Case studies are used to illustrate the author's ideas.

I. COMPREHENSIVE RESOURCE GUIDES

Each of these selections contains extensive resource listings that can supplement the individual resources we have provided. A thorough listing of agencies, organizations, consumer groups, books, and materials is provided by each of these excellent handbooks of resources for disabled individuals and their families.

1. Moore, C., Gorham-Morton, K., & Southard, A. (1983). *A reader's guide for parents of children with mental, physical or emotional disabilities.* Baltimore: Maryland State Planning Council on Developmental Disabilities. $15.95.

   This book, written for parents of disabled and chronically ill children, provides annotated bibliographies of books and resources. A variety of disabilities and illnesses are specifically addressed (e.g., autism, emotional disability, epilepsy, hearing and visual impairment, hyperactivity, learning disabilities, and mental retardation) in six categories: basic reading, personal accounts, the early years, school years, when children become adults, and where to write for information. In addition, a number of topics of special interest are covered, such as attitudes, behavior modification, death and dying, genetic counseling, future planning, the rights of children, and sexuality. Finally, an extensive index provides information on organizations, directories, journals, and more.

2. Katz, A. H., & Martin, K. (1982). *A handbook of services for the handicapped.* Westport, CT: Greenwood Press. $35.00.

   This handbook provides an excellent and comprehensive resource of the many services available to disabled individuals of all ages. Chapters cover physical care, housing, financial aid, employment, vocational rehabilitation, counseling, recreation and social activities, and special services for children. Each chapter provides extremely valuable and detailed information about these services. For example, the financial aid chapter covers the goals and eligibility requirements for unemployment, long-term disability, old age, aid to families with dependent children, housing, veterans and workers compensation, food stamps, and more. An appendix also provides an extensive listing of national advocacy, consumer, and voluntary organizations. This book is a useful, intelligent guide to families seeking to resolve disability-related needs.

3. Ecumenical Task Force on the Church and the Disabled. (1982). *A resource manual for full participation.* Madison, WI: Author. $18.95.

    This handbook was compiled to help religious and community leaders integrate people with disabilities into their communities of faith. Included are both practical suggestions for relating and ministering to the disabled, as well as information about stereotypes, discrimination, and common myths. In addition to containing suggestions for implementation and accessibility, this handbook provides an extensive listing of resources, including national and state organizations, audiovisual resources, recreational resources, educational and religious resources, and books and materials for children with a range of specific disabilities. This resource manual can help ensure successful interaction between families with disabled members and the church or synagogue of their choice. *Contact:* Wisconsin Conference of Churches, 1955 W. Broadway, Madison, WI 53173 (608) 222-9779.

J. Organizations

Some organizations that may be able to provide you with information are listed below. For information on additional organizations, you might want to refer to one of the comprehensive resource guides listed in the previous section.

American Association on Mental Deficiency (AAMD), 1719 Kalorama Road, N.W., Washington, DC 20009.

American Cancer Society, 777 3rd Avenue, New York, NY 10017.

American Council of the Blind, 1211 Connecticut Avenue, N.W., Suite 506, Washington, DC 20036.

American Diabetes Association, 600 Fifth Avenue, New York, NY 10020.

American Heart Association, 7320 Greenville Avenue, Dallas, TX 75231.

American Parkinson Disease Association, 147 East 50th Street, New York, NY 10022.

Arthritis Foundation, 3400 Peachtree Road, N.E., Suite 1101, Atlanta, GA 30326.

Association for Children and Adults with Learning Disabilities, 4156 Library Road, Pittsburgh, PA 15234.

Association for Retarded Citizens (ARC), 2501 Avenue J, Arlington, TX 76011.

Asthma and Allergy Foundation of America, 19 West 44th Street, New York, NY 10036.

Closer Look (information for parents of children with disabilities), Box 1492, Washington, DC 20013.

Council for Exceptional Children, 1920 Association Drive, Reston, VA 22091.

Cystic Fibrosis Foundation, 6000 Executive Boulevard, Suite 309, Rockville, MD 20852.

Epilepsy Foundation of America, 4351 Garden City Drive, Landover, MD 29781.

International Association of Parents of the Deaf (IAPD), 814 Thayer Avenue, Silver Spring, MD 20910.

Leukemia Society of America, 800 Second Avenue, New York, NY 10017.

March of Dimes Birth Defects Foundation, 1275 Mamaroneck Avenue, White Plains, NY 10605.

Mental Health Association, 1800 North Kent Street, Arlington, VA 22209.

Muscular Dystrophy Association, 810 Seventh Avenue, New York, NY 10019.

National Association for Independent Living, 1599 Case Road, Columbus, OH 43224.

National Association for the Deaf, 814 Thayer Avenue, Silver Spring, MD 20910.

National Association for the Deaf-Blind, 2703 Forest Oak Circle, Norman, OK 73071.

National Easter Seal Society, 2023 West Ogden Avenue, Chicago, IL 60612.

National Head Injury Foundation, 280 Singletary Lane, Framingham, MA 01701.

National Huntington's Disease Association, 128-A East 74th Street, New York, NY 10021.

National Information Center for Handicapped Youth and Children, P.O. Box 1492, Washington, DC 20013.

National Kidney Foundation, 2 Park Avenue, New York, NY 10016.

National Mental Health Association National Headquarters, 1800 North Kent Street, Rosslyn, VA 22209.

National Multiple Sclerosis Society, 205 East 80th Street, New York, NY 10017.

The National Society for Children and Adults with Autism (NSAC), 1234 Massachusetts Avenue, N.W., Suite 1017, Washington, DC 20005-4599.

National Spinal Cord Injury Association, 369 Elliot Street, Newton Upper Falls, MA 02164.

Spina Bifida Association of America, 343 South Dearborn Avenue, Suite 319, Chicago, IL 60604.

The Association for Persons with Severe Handicaps (TASH), 7010 Roosevelt Way, N.E., Seattle, WA 98115.

United Cerebral Palsy Associations, 66 East 34th Street, New York, NY 10016.

United Ostomy Association, 2001 West Beverly Boulevard, Los Angeles, CA 90057.

United Parkinson Foundation, 360 West Superior Street, Chicago, IL 60610.

References

Brotherson, M. J., Backus, L. H., Summers, J. A., & Turnbull, A. P. (1986). Transition to adulthood. In J. A. Summers (Ed.), *The right to grow up: An introduction to adults with developmental disabilities.* Baltimore: Paul H. Brookes Publishing Co.

Cobb, S. (1976). Social support as a mediator of life stress. *Journal of Psychosomatic Medicine, 38,* 300–314.

Diamond, S. (1981). Growing up with parents of a handicapped child: A handicapped person's perspective. In J. L. Paul (Ed.), *Understanding and working with parents of children with special needs.* New York: Holt, Rinehart, & Winston.

Lyons, S., & Preis, A. (1983). Working with families of severely handicapped persons. In M. Seligman (Ed.), *The family with a handicapped child: Understanding and treatment.* New York: Grune & Stratton.

Rubin, S., & Quinn-Curran, N. (1983). Lost, then found: Parents' journey through the community service maze. In M. Seligman (Ed.), *The family with a handicapped child: Understanding and treatment.* New York: Grune & Stratton.

Index

Exercises

In order to allow your family more flexibility in completing the exercises discussed in each chapter, the following pages have been perforated and can be torn out of the book. These exercises were designed for you to complete in the most convenient manner possible, individually or as a group.

1. List the *three* values that are *most* important to you in life. (Use Table 2.1 (on page 19) to help you get started in your thinking, but of course, don't limit yourself—what's most important to *you* ?)

2. Compare your answers with those of other family members. How are they similar? Different? How do all your family values affect the way you live?

3. If possible, think about your life before there was a disability or illness in your family. What were your top values then? How has the disability or illness affected your family's values?

Exercise 2B

1. Think of a stressful event that happened to you within the last 6 months. What did you do to cope with the stress?

2. Ask other family members or friends to think of a stressful event and how they coped. Make a list of the different coping strategies suggested.

3. Think of alternative coping strategies you could have used to deal with your stress. Which strategies would you like to use more in the future? Which less?

Exercise 3A

1. List everyone whom you consider to be a part of your family.

2. List other relatives, close friends, neighbors, co-workers, church or synagogue members, and others who provide you with social support.

3. Listed below are several types of people who might make up your social support network, along with a scale to rate how helpful they are. Circle the number that best describes how helpful each one is to you. Leave the space blank if that person or group does not apply to you. Use a different color pen for each family member who fills this out, and compare your answers.

Family support scale

	Not at all helpful	Some-times helpful	Gener-ally helpful	Very helpful	Extremely helpful
1. My parents	0	1	2	3	4
2. My spouse's parents	0	1	2	3	4
3. My relatives/kin	0	1	2	3	4
4. My spouse's relatives/ kin	0	1	2	3	4
5. Husband or wife	0	1	2	3	4
6. My friends	0	1	2	3	4
7. My spouse's friends	0	1	2	3	4
8. My own children	0	1	2	3	4
9. Other parents	0	1	2	3	4
10. My family physician	0	1	2	3	4

(continued)

Exercise 3A

(continued)

Family support scale

		Not at all helpful	Some-times helpful	Gener-ally helpful	Very helpful	Extremely helpful
11.	Co-workers	0	1	2	3	4
12.	Parent, spouse, or other self-help groups	0	1	2	3	4
13.	School (teachers, therapists, psychologists, etc.)	0	1	2	3	4
14.	Professional agencies (public health, social services, respite care, activity programs)	0	1	2	3	4
15.	Civic groups/clubs	0	1	2	3	4
16.	Clergy and congregation of your place of worship	0	1	2	3	4

Exercise 3B

1. Think about the roadblocks that you have to using friends, neighbors, and relatives for social support. We have listed a few in the text (see pages 33–37) but include any others that are specific to your family.

2. Now divide those roadblocks into two groups: those that are practical roadblocks, such as lack of time or transportation, and those that are value roadblocks, such as believing you have sole responsibility or that you do not want to burden others. List your roadblocks under each category.

   Practical roadblocks   **Value roadblocks**

3. Select one roadblock from each group, and list steps you could use to overcome that roadblock. Discuss your steps with other family members.

   Practical roadblock   **Value roadblock**

   _____   _____

   Steps: Steps:

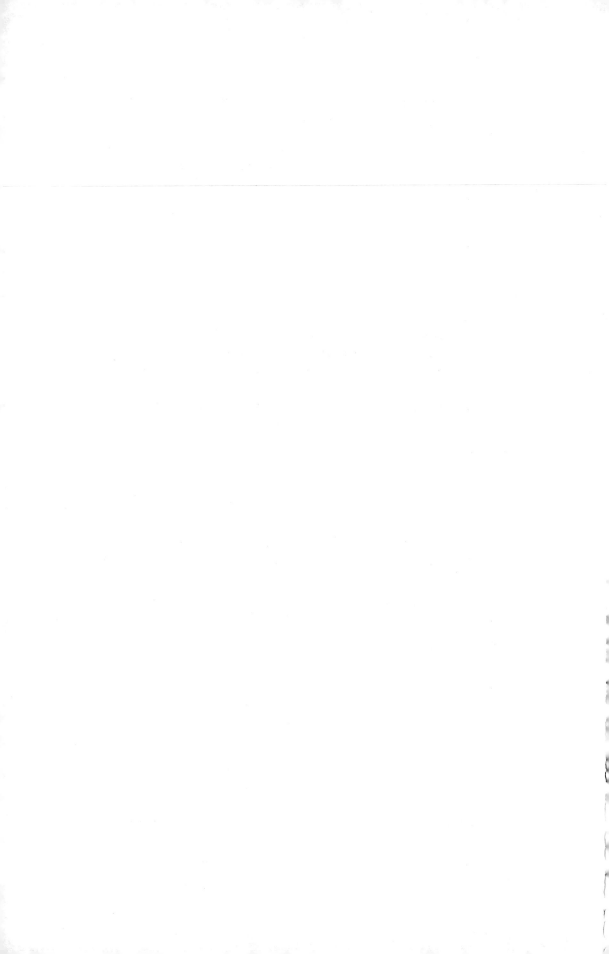

Exercise 4A

1. Think of a professional who has been particularly helpful to you. List some of the things that made the experience successful for you.

2. Think of a professional who was particularly *unhelpful* to you. List what was unhelpful about him or her. In retrospect, is there some way you could have handled the interaction differently?

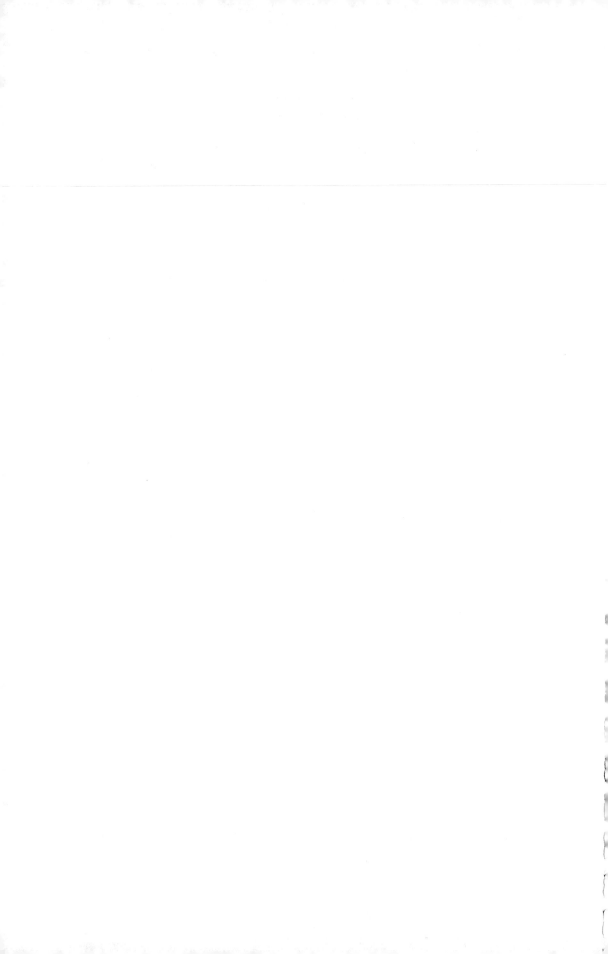

Exercise 4B

1. List the roadblocks you have experienced in using professional support. We have listed a few, but include any others your family has encountered.

2. Select one roadblock and list possible ways to overcome that roadblock. Discuss your ideas with other family members.

Exercise 5A

Below is a list of needs common to most families, organized within each of the eight basic areas of need. We have left some blanks in each area for you to add any other needs that might be special to your family. First, consider how important each need is to YOU. Rate each one in Column A on a scale of 0—4 as follows:

0	1	2	3	4
not applicable	not important at all	a little important	somewhat important	very important

Second, consider how fully you believe each need is being met. In Column B, rate each one in terms of your satisfaction with the degree to which it is met on a scale of 0—4 as follows:

0	1	2	3	4
not applicable	very unsatisfied	usually unsatisfied	usually satisfied	very satisfied

Column A   Column B

Economic
Making enough money
Having a good job
Managing the budget
Teaching children about money
Other:
_____
_____

Health and Security
Exercising
Eating right
Getting enough rest
Getting enough medical and
   dental care
Feeling free from danger
Other:
_____
_____

Physical
Cooking and eating meals
Taking care of clothes (laundry,
   mending, ironing, etc.)
Taking care of yourself (bathing,
   dressing, grooming, etc.)
Cleaning house
Having adequate transportation
Shopping
Making household repairs
Doing yard work
Other:
_____
_____

(continued)

	Column A	Column B

Recreation

Having interesting hobbies
Participating in sports
Having family fun
Just relaxing
Other:

_____

_____

Socialization

Being with family
Being with friends
Having close friends
Other:

_____

_____

Self-Definition

Knowing yourself
Feeling needed and worthwhile
Feeling content with who you are
Needing other people
Feeling good about job
Feeling good about home and
   family
Other:

_____

_____

Affection

Feeling loved
Expressing love
Having intimate relationships
Feeling satisfied with sexual
   intimacy
Other:

_____

_____

Education

Going to school (school,
   college, technical, etc.)
Learning new job skills
Learning new things in general
Other:

_____

_____

Exercise 5B

Below is a list of tasks commonly associated with meeting the needs listed in Exercise 5A. We have left some blanks for you to add any other tasks that are special to your family. You may also want to put "NA" beside any tasks your family does not do. In Column A, write the names or initials of ALL the members of your family who do these tasks. In Column B, write the names or initials of friends, neighbors, relatives, co-workers, or other people who help out with each task. Finally, in Column C, write the names or initials of any service agencies or professionals who provide help in that area. You might want to look back at Exercise 3A to jog your memory about the various people who make up your social and professional network.

	Column A (Family members)	Column B (Social support)	Column C (Professional support)

Economic
Making money
Managing the budget
Teaching children about money
Other:

_____

_____

Health and Security
Teaching children
   about diet and exercise
Providing medical,
   dental, and eye care
Providing security
Other:

_____

_____

Physical
Cooking and cleaning up
Cleaning house
Taking care of clothes
   (laundry, mending, etc.)
Grooming (bathing,
   dressing, etc.) small children,
   disabled or ill person
Driving and maintaining car
Shopping
Fixing things around the house
Doing yard work
Other:

_____

_____

Recreation
Helping other family
   members with hobbies
Playing games or sports
   with other family members
Going on or organizing outings
Relaxing around the
   house with family
Other:

_____

_____

(continued)

	Column A	Column B	Column C

Socialization

Teaching family members
  to interact with others
Spending time with friends
Spending time with
  other family members
Talking/listening to others
Other:

_____

_____

Self-Definition

Expressing appreciation
  to other family members
Supporting other family
  members in their jobs
Supporting other
  family members in
  their role at home
Providing constructive
  feedback to other
  family members
Other:

_____

_____

Affection

Expressing affection
Expressing personal
  feelings to others
Initiating intimacy
Other:

_____

_____

Education

Helping other family
  members with homework
Supporting other family
  members in their education
Teaching skills to
  others (for example,
  cooking, car repair)
Teaching religious
  and/or other values
Teaching general
  knowledge to others
Other:

_____

_____

Below we have provided spaces for each of the eight broad areas of family needs. In the first column, think of people in your social support network (friends, relatives, neighbors, co-workers, etc.) who could be helpful in that area. Beside their names, jot down the specific way they can help. Do the same thing in the second column for professionals or agencies in your community. In both cases, try to think of people or agencies you did NOT include in that particular area of need in Exercise 5B. In other words, try to think of resources you are not using now. For example, one family had an aunt and uncle who lived nearby and a city recreation department. Their list of ways these supports could be helpful in the area of recreation is included as an example.

Recreation

Social supporters   Professional supporters

Aunt Helen—can take Joey   *Rec. Dept.—we can enroll Joey*
    to the park   *in swimming class*

Economic needs

Social supporters   Professional supporters

Health and security needs

Social supporters   Professional supporters

Physical needs

Social supporters   Professional supporters

(continued)

Exercise 5C
(continued)

Recreational needs

Social supporters   Professional supporters

Socialization needs

Social supporters   Professional supporters

Self-definition needs

Social supporters   Professional supporters

Affectional needs

Social supporters   Professional supporters

Educational needs

Social supporters   Professional supporters

Exercise 6A

1. Recall a situation in which you felt particularly let down and disappointed after having discussed a concern or problem with someone.

   What did the person say that disappointed you?

   _____

   What didn't he or she say?

   _____

   What was most unhelpful about the interaction?

   _____

   How might you have contributed to this unhelpful experience?

   _____

   What would you do differently in the future?

   _____

   How did you feel about the problem afterwards?

   _____

2. Now think of a situation in which you felt particularly pleased and assisted by another person with whom you discussed a problem or concern.

   What did the person do or say that made communication clear and easy?

   _____

   What was most helpful about his or her manner or response?

   _____

   What did you do to contribute to the success of this interaction?

   _____

   How did you feel about the problem afterwards?

   _____

Exercise 6B

Consider the following example:

> Joyce Wethers is a single mother whose 3-year-old son James has been diagnosed as autistic. For weeks, Joyce has been trying to locate a satisfactory educational program for James, but to no avail. Despite numerous telephone calls, Joyce feels that she has gotten the "runaround," and she wonders if there is any justice at all for children with disabilities. Frustrated and angry, Joyce decides to contact the superintendent of the public school system directly, both to express her need and to attain some assistance. Before picking up the receiver, she pauses and considers what to say.

How might Joyce best communicate her needs and concerns to the superintendent? Put yourself in Joyce's place, and write what you would say:

_____

_____

_____

_____

Below, check the styles of communication you incorporated into your message:

_____ Used more heart than mind
_____ Used more mind than heart
_____ Used equal balance of heart and mind
_____ Assumed responsibility
_____ Imposed blame
_____ Included threats
_____ Straightforwardness
_____ Presented calmly
_____ Avoided mind reading
_____ Will likely build communication (would be constructive if spoken to me)

What were the best aspects of your message?

_____

_____

What aspects of your message would you change?

_____

_____

Exercise 6C

1. How do you feel others know that you are paying attention? How successful do you feel you are in letting others know that they are being heard?

2. Ask another family member the following questions:
   a. How well do you feel I pay attention to you when you speak?

   b. How do you know that I am paying attention (what signs do I give you)?

3. What did you learn about your listening skills? List below those aspects that you would like to change or emphasize even more:

   _____   _____
   _____   _____
   _____   _____
   _____   _____
   _____   _____
   _____   _____
   _____   _____
   _____   _____

Exercise 6D

Assume that the following messages are directed at you. As an active listener, paraphrase each message in order to check out your understanding.

Example: "Don will never be able to take care of himself—his future is hopeless."

Response: "It sounds like you are feeling hopeless about Don's future."

Message 1: "I just can't do it all on my own anymore. I just can't stand it!"

Response 1:

Message 2: "Our sex life is nonexistent. You must not really love me anymore."

Response 2:

Message 3: "Nobody cares what I want. I might as well not even be part of a family."

Response 3:

Exercise 7A

Think of a need you have been aware of during the past month. List three destructive need statements and then three constructive need statements to convey that need. Choose the best statement and try it out on a family member. How did he or she react?

NEED:

Three destructive need statements:

1. _____
   _____
2. _____
   _____
3. _____
   _____

Three constructive need statements:

1. _____
   _____
2. _____
   _____
3. _____
   _____

Best statement:

Exercise 7B

Gather your family together, picking a time that is most comfortable for everyone. Have each member take a turn expressing two unmet needs he or she is currently experiencing within the family. Express each need with an "I" statement, specifying the nature of the need and without attributing blame or responsibility to others. Similarly, try to listen to each other without defensiveness or argument. (If you can't think of any unmet needs, refer to the checklist you completed in Chapter 5.)

Finally, paraphrase each member's need statements in a constructive manner in order to check out the accuracy of the family's understanding. Have one member record each need statement and the accompanying paraphrased response in the spaces provided. Here are three examples of need statements and paraphrased responses:

Need Statement: I need to feel less overwhelmed by all the demands on my time and energy.

Paraphrase: You seem to feel like it's hard for you to set priorities for everything you feel like you need to do.

Need Statement: I hate to take my pills everyday.

Paraphrase: It sounds like you are really feeling how hard it is to live with an illness.

Need Statement: I need more money from somewhere to pay for the medicine and equipment I need.

Paraphrase: Maybe we could all put our heads together and try to figure out better ways to get your health-related needs paid for.

1. Need statement: _____

   Paraphrase: _____

2. Need statement: _____

   Paraphrase: _____

3. Need statement: _____

   Paraphrase: _____

(continued)

Exercise 7B
(continued)

4. Need statement: _____

    _____

    Paraphrase: _____

    _____

5. Need statement: _____

    _____

    Paraphrase: _____

    _____

6. Need statement: _____

    _____

    Paraphrase: _____

    _____

Exercise 7C

Look over the list of need statements generated by family members in Exercise 7B. Select two for each family member, and restate each one as a solvable problem definition. That is, state each one in such a way that solutions are not included in the definition and specific actions comprise the focus of the statement. Save a copy of these problem definitions for later use. Here are some sample need statements and accompanying solvable problem definitions:

Need Statement	Solvable Problem Definition
Example A: I need more money for medicine and equipment.	I need a plan to figure out how I can get the medicine and equipment I need.
Example B: I need to feel less overwhelmed by work.	I need to find ways to arrange by priority everything I need to do so I can cope with it all.

1. _____ _____

2. _____ _____

3. _____ _____

4. _____ _____

5. _____ _____

6. _____ _____

Look back at the list of problem definitions you developed in Exercise 7C. Put a "U" beside each one that you think is unrelated to your family member's illness or disability. For example, a family might decide that a problem defined as obtaining better financial opportunities is not related to illness or disability. Put an "R" beside those problems that you think are primarily caused by the special need; for example, alleviating a family member's depression following a traumatic accident. Third, put a "B" beside those problems that involve issues both related and unrelated to the special need of an ill or disabled family member.

Next, choose *two* of the problems from your list, and see if you can differentiate which aspects of each relate to the special need and which do not. Here are two examples:

Example 1:

Problem definition: Determine vocational choice for an adolescent with paraplegia. **B**

Disability-related issues: 1) physical limitations, 2) accessible location, 3) overcoming potential discrimination

Non-disability-related issues: 1) preferences and goals, 2) self-concept and confidence, 3) fears

Example 2 (from Exercise 7C, Example A):

Problem definition: I need a plan to figure out how to get money for the equipment I need. **B**

Disability-related issues: Need medication, equipment, resources depleted by other disability-related needs

Non-disability-related issues: Economically disadvantaged, anger at system, preference to spend money on other things

1. *Problem definition:* _____
   _____
   _____

   Disability-related issues: _____
   _____
   _____

   Non-disability-related issues: _____
   _____
   _____

(continued)

Exercise 7D
(continued)

2. *Problem definition:* _____

     _____

     _____

     Disability-related issues: _____

     _____

     _____

     Non-disability-related issues: _____

     _____

     _____

Exercise 7E

List three problems that have recently or in the past seemed unsolvable. Spend a few minutes thinking of aspects of each problem that you can control, manage, and change. Do these aspects seem easier to target for resolution than the problems you first listed?

"Unsolvable" Problems	**Controllable Aspects**
1.	a.
	b.
	c.
	d.
2.	a.
	b.
	c.
	d.
3.	a.
	b.
	c.
	d.

Exercise 7F

Look back at the six case studies in Chapter 1 and choose one family. Pretend that this family has asked yours to tell them which of their many problems they need to work on first. Either individually or as a group, think of criteria you deem important for selecting a problem to address.

List them briefly:

1. _____ _____
2. _____ _____
3. _____ _____
4. _____ _____
5. _____ _____
6. _____ _____
7. _____ _____
8. _____ _____
9. _____ _____
10. _____ _____

Talk over your criteria as a family, and try to reach agreement on the five most important criteria. Put a "1" through "5" beside each one of these, in order of importance.

Now, look at the problem definitions for your own family in Exercise 7C, and try to use the criteria you just listed to select one problem to address. Briefly state each problem definition in the spaces on the left-hand side of the worksheet below. Then, think whether your first problem meets criterion number 1; if it does, put a check (√) in the box. Do the same with criteria numbers 2–5. Continue in this way until you have rated all your problem definitions. Talk over your answers with each other. Can you reach agreement on a problem to solve first? (If you need more room, do this exercise on a separate sheet.)

Problems	Criteria				
	1	2	3	4	5
1. _____	☐	☐	☐	☐	☐
2. _____	☐	☐	☐	☐	☐
3. _____	☐	☐	☐	☐	☐
4. _____	☐	☐	☐	☐	☐
5. _____	☐	☐	☐	☐	☐
6. _____	☐	☐	☐	☐	☐

Exercise 8A

Using one problem identified in Chapter 7, work through the following three steps in order to determine whom to involve in the brainstorming process.

Step 1: List your family members and any possible friends, community people, or professionals who may be helpful in solving this problem. You may want to refer to your inventory of social and professional support in Chapter 3 (Exercise 3A).

1.	9.
2.	10.
3.	11.
4.	12.
5.	13.
6.	14.
7.	15.
8.	16.

Step 2: Which issues are important to consider concerning whom to involve in decision making? We have provided a few, but add your own to the list. Determine whether each potential participant meets each of the criteria on your list.

1. Affected by problem?
2. Wants to participate?
3. Has expertise?
4. Provides different perspective?
5. Creative?
6. _____
7. _____
8. _____
9. _____
10. _____
11. _____
12. _____

Step 3: Briefly list whom you decided to involve and why. If someone you want to include has not met many of the criteria, explain why you still want to involve him or her (e.g., his opinion is important to us; she is caring and honest; he is willing to contribute).

Exercise 8B

Consider the following case study:

> Matt and Nina Galanto have been married for 5 years. Since Matt suffered a spinal cord injury 1 year after their marriage, both have had to make a number of adjustments. Nina has taken on much of the financial responsibility, working as a typist, while Matt is employed part-time as a math tutor.
>
> Matt has tried to adjust to a greater degree of dependence on Nina than he finds comfortable. Particularly troubling to Matt is his wife's constant involvement in many of his personal care needs. On the one hand, Matt feels that he needs help bathing, dressing, and so forth, and appreciates Nina's help. Yet, on the other hand, he has come to resent his dependence and finds her help intrusive and embarrassing. Similarly, although Nina feels responsible for helping Matt, she is finding that the physical strain and constant tension are taking their toll on her as well. As a result, Matt and Nina have defined a problem: Matt and Nina need greater independence from each other, primarily in terms of Matt's personal care needs.

What alternatives might the Galantos consider to resolve their current problem? As a family, generate as many alternatives as possible for the Galantos' situation. Write them down on a separate piece of paper or below. Try to make sure each participant contributes at least one idea. (*Note:* If you feel you don't have enough facts about this family to generate many solutions, invent the facts! The idea of this exercise is for your family to practice being as creative as possible.)

Exercise 8C

Convene as many of the brainstorming participants you identified in Exercise 8A as possible. Choose a current family problem—for example one identified in a previous exercise—and begin to brainstorm alternative means of satisfying that need. Everyone involved should be encouraged to contribute ideas. Be careful not to censor your own or other members' ideas or to evaluate their suggestions in any way. In other words, emphasize creativity; suggest seemingly unusual ideas. Children can be encouraged to contribute their ideas particularly well in a nonjudgmental and open brainstorming session. Their imagination and lack of inhibitions may spark many new ideas with a little added encouragement and reinforcement. Record a list of all the alternatives generated by your family on a separate sheet of paper or below. (Be sure to save it for use in the exercises in the next chapter.) Talk to anyone who was unable to attend the brainstorming session, and add their ideas to your list.

Exercise 9A

Using the list obtained from your brainstorming exercise in Chapter 8, gather the family together for an evaluation session. If this is not convenient, each person could do this exercise separately and compare results later. On the back of this page, Worksheet 9A, which is similar to Table 9.1 (on pages 136–137) in which Mary and Tom Jones evaluated their alternatives, is blank. Put your own problem statement (from Chapter 7) at the top of the page and brief descriptions of each of your brainstormed alternatives down the side. If you are doing this exercise as a group, have one member read each alternative, and then decide together to which category it belongs. Record your answers in the table. Encourage everyone in the family to participate, and include a "why" statement along with each decision. Practice accepting others' opinions as helpful input, avoiding criticism or argument. When differences of opinion do arise, use the negotiation and communication skills you have acquired to resolve them.

Worksheet 9A. Assigning alternatives to categories

Alternatives	Categories			Why statements
	Avoids problems	Demands that only one change	Cooperation and negotiation	

Exercise 9B

On the back of this page, Worksheet 9B is a worksheet similar to the one used by the Changs (see page 142). List those alternatives from Exercise 9A that involve cooperation and negotiation down the side of the table. Now you are ready to evaluate them.

Step 1: Think about the possible outcomes of each alternative. This is best done as a group—discuss together what you think would happen if each alternative was employed.

Step 2: Have each family member rate each alternative with a plus or a minus.

Step 3: For each alternative, score an overall "plus" in the total column if the majority of the group gives it a "plus." Give the alternative a "minus" if the majority of the group does not like the alternative. Using communication skills, discuss and negotiate alternatives with tied scores.

Worksheet 9B. Evaluating alternatives

Alternatives	Possible outcomes	Family member ratings	Overall rating

Exercise 9C

Worksheet 9C, on the back of this page, is a blank worksheet arranged similarly to the one used by the Chang family (see page 144) in completing this exercise.

Step One: As a family, think of all the possible results of a *perfect* solution to the problem you are addressing. To provide clues, refer to your family values (Chapter 2) and the needs you consider most important (Chapter 5). Put these criteria in the space provided on the worksheet.

Step Two: Look back at your answers in Exercise 9B, and list all the alternatives receiving an overall "plus" rating across the top of the page.

Step Three: Consider which criteria each alternative meets. Place an "X" in the box where the alternative meets the criterion.

Step Four: Put the total number of criteria met by each alternative at the bottom of the page.

Worksheet 9C. Using criteria to evaluate alternatives

Criteria	Alternatives					
Total number of criteria met:						

Exercise 9D

Using the criteria worksheet completed in Exercise 9C, compare the criteria (and criteria totals) met by each alternative. Does one stand out as superior to the others? If so, are family members in agreement that this is the best alternative? If no one alternative is clearly the best one, discuss which alternative seems to meet the most important criteria. Employ negotiation and communication skills to exchange ideas, work through differences, and arrive at a decision that is acceptable to the majority of those family members involved in the problem-solving process. The end result should be a chosen plan of attack in resolving a current family problem.

Exercise 10A

Using the solution your family chose to resolve a family problem in Exercise 9D, complete the following steps:

Step 1: Discuss and specify steps of the solution that need further planning.

Step 2: Brainstorm alternative plans for implementing each step of the plan.

Step 3: Evaluate each alternative by discussion and/or ratings. Negotiate a mutually agreeable plan for each phase of the solution.

Exercise 10B

Using your step-by-step plan mapped out in Exercise 10A, assemble the family and assign responsibility for steps within the plan to individual family members. During the entire procedure, pay careful attention to communication patterns within the family. As individuals, ask the following questions: How are conflicts handled? Does one person dominate discussion or remain conspicuously quiet? Are differences of opinion negotiated to a satisfactory compromise? Is each person satisfied with the task assignments? Discuss your individual answers to these questions as a family.